T0362120

Adolescent Health in the Covid-19 Post-Pandemic

Editors

RENATA ARRINGTON-SANDERS
ERROL L. FIELDS

PEDIATRIC CLINICS OF NORTH AMERICA

www.pediatric.theclinics.com

Consulting Editor
TINA L. CHENG

August 2024 • Volume 71 • Number 4

ELSEVIER

1600 John F. Kennedy Boulevard ● Suite 1800 ● Philadelphia, Pennsylvania, 19103-2899

http://www.theclinics.com

THE PEDIATRIC CLINICS OF NORTH AMERICA Volume 71, Number 4
August 2024 ISSN 0031-3955, ISBN-13: 978-0-443-12907-0

Editor: Kerry Holland
Developmental Editor: Saswoti Nath

The Pediatric Clinics of North America (ISSN 0031-3955) is published bimonthly by Elsevier Inc., 360 Park Avenue South, New York, NY 10010-1710. Months of issue are February, April, June, August, October, and December. Periodicals postage paid at New York, NY and additional mailing offices. Subscription prices are $290.00 per year (US individuals), $368.00 per year (Canadian individuals), $440.00 per year (international individuals), $100.00 per year (US students and residents), $100.00 per year (Canadian students and residents), and $165.00 per year (international residents and students). For institutional access pricing please contact Customer Service via the contact information below. To receive students/resident rare, orders must be accompanied by name of affiliated institution, date of term, and the signature of program/residency coordinator on institution letterhead. Orders will be billed at individual rate until proof of status is received. Foreign air speed delivery is included in all *Clinics* subscription prices. All prices are subject to change without notice. **POSTMASTER:** Send address changes to *The Pediatric Clinics of North America*, Elsevier Health Sciences Division, Subscription Customer Service, 3251 Riverport Lane, Maryland Heights, MO 63043. **Customer Service: 1-800-654-2452 (US and Canada). From outside of the US and Canada: 1-314-447-8871. Fax: 1-314-447-8029. For print support, E-mail: JournalsCustomerService-usa@elsevier.com. For online support, E-mail: JournalsOnlineSupport-usa@elsevier.com.**

Reprints. For copies of 100 or more, of articles in this publication, please contact the Commercial Reprints Department, Elsevier Inc., 360 Park Avenue South, New York, NY 10010-1710. Tel.: 212-633-3874; Fax: 212-633-3820; E-mail: reprints@elsevier.com.

The Pediatric Clinics of North America is also published in Spanish by McGraw-Hill Inter-americana Editores S.A., Mexico City, Mexico; in Portuguese by Riechmann and Affonso Editores, Rua Comandante Coelho 1085, CEP 21250, Rio de Janeiro, Brazil; and in Greek by Althayia SA, Athens, Greece.

The Pediatric Clinics of North America is covered in *MEDLINE/PubMed (Index Medicus), Excerpta Medica, Current Contents, Current Contents/Clinical Medicine, Science Citation Index, ASCA, ISI/BIOMED,* and *BIOSIS.*

Contributors

CONSULTING EDITOR

TINA L. CHENG, MD, MPH
BK Rachford Professor and Chair of Pediatrics, University of Cincinnati, Director, Cincinnati Children's Research Foundation, Chief Medical Officer, Cincinnati Children's Hospital Medical Center, Cincinnati, Ohio, USA

EDITORS

RENATA ARRINGTON-SANDERS, MD, MPH, ScM
Chief, Craig-Dalsimer Division of Adolescent Medicine, Professor of Pediatrics and Medicine, Orton Jackson Endowed Chair in Adolescent Medicine, Perelman School of Medicine, University of Pennsylvania, The Children's Hospital of Philadelphia, Pennsylvania, USA

ERROL L. FIELDS, MD, PhD, MPH
Associate Professor of Pediatrics, Division of Adolescent and Young Adult Medicine, Johns Hopkins School of Medicine, Baltimore, Maryland

AUTHORS

HOOVER ADGER, MD, MPH, MBA
Division of Adolescent and Young Adult Medicine, Department of Pediatrics, Johns Hopkins University School of Medicine, Baltimore, Maryland, USA

SUZANNE ALLEN, MSN, CPNP
Instructor of Pediatrics, University of Massachusetts Memorial Children's Medical Center, UMass Chan Medical School, Tan Chingfen Graduate School of Nursing, Worcester, Massachusetts, USA

RENATA ARRINGTON-SANDERS, MD, MPH, ScM
Chief, Craig-Dalsimer Division of Adolescent Medicine, Professor of Pediatrics and Medicine, Orton Jackson Endowed Chair in Adolescent Medicine, Perelman School of Medicine, University of Pennsylvania, The Children's Hospital of Philadelphia, Pennsylvania, USA

SARAH H. ARSHAD, MD
Assistant Professor of Clinical Psychiatry, Children's Hospital of Philadelphia, University of Pennsylvania Perelman School of Medicine, Philadelphia, Pennsylvania, USA

ALBA AZOLA, MD
Assistant Professor, Department of Pediatrics, Division of Adolescent and Young Adult Medicine, Assistant Professor, Department of Physical Medicine and Rehabilitation, Johns Hopkins School of Medicine, Baltimore, Maryland, USA

JESSE BARONDEAU, MD
Division Chief, Adolescent Medicine, Assistant Professor, Division of Adolescent Medicine, University of Nebraska, College of Medicine, University of Nebraska Medical Center, Children's Nebraska, Omaha, Nebraska, USA

TAMI D. BENTON, MD
Psychiatrist-in-Chief, Frederick H. Allen Endowed Chair in Child Psychiatry Chair, Director of Education, Department of Child and Adolescent Psychiatry and Behavioral Sciences, Children's Hospital of Philadelphia, Professor of Clinical Psychiatry and Pediatrics, Perelman School of Medicine at the University of Pennsylvania, Philadelphia, Pennsylvania, USA

DEBRA BRAUN-COURVILLE, MD
Assistant Professor, Department of Pediatrics, Division of Adolescent and Young Adult Health, Vanderbilt University Medical Center, Nashville, Tennessee, USA

MERRIAN J. BROOKS, DO, MS
Attending Pediatrician, Adolescent Medicine Specialist, Craig Dalsimer Division of Adolescent Medicine, Children's Hospital of Philadelphia, Assistant Professor, Department of Pediatrics, University of Pennsylvania Perelman School of Medicine, Philadelphia, Pennsylvania, USA; Lead Pediatrician Botswana UPENN Partnership, Gaborone, Botswana

CAMILLE A. BROUSSARD, MD, MPH
Assistant Professor, Department of Pediatrics, Division of Adolescent and Young Adult Medicine, Johns Hopkins School of Medicine, Baltimore, Maryland, USA

JOANNA BROWN, MD, MPH
Attending Physician, Division of Adolescent and Young Adult Medicine, Boston Children's Hospital, Boston, Massachusetts, USA

ELVIRA CHICCARELLI, MD
Assistant Professor of Pediatrics, Uniformed Services University of the Health Sciences, Brooke Army Medical Center, Fort Sam Houston, Texas, USA

JEYLAN CLOSE, MD
Medical Instructor, National Clinician Scholars Program, Department of Psychiatry and Behavioral Sciences, Child and Family Mental Health and Community Psychiatry Division, Duke University School of Medicine, Duke Margolis Center for Health Policy, Duke University, Durham, North Carolina, USA

LAKESHIA N. CRAIG, MD
Assistant Professor, Department of Pediatrics, Division of Adolescent Medicine, Medical University of South Carolina, College of Medicine, North Charleston, South Carolina, USA

ALISON CULYBA, MD, PhD, MPH
Director, Division of Adolescent and Young Adult Medicine, Associate Professor of Pediatrics, Public Health, and Clinical and Translational Science, University of Pittsburgh School of Medicine, UPMC Children's Hospital of Pittsburgh, Pittsburgh, Pennsylvania, USA

STEPHANIE DAVIDSON, MD
Assistant Professor of Clinical Psychiatry, Perelman School of Medicine at the University of Pennsylvania, Department of Child and Adolescent Psychiatry and Behavioral Sciences, Children's Hospital of Philadelphia, Philadelphia, Pennsylvania, USA

NEERAV DESAI, MD
Associate Professor, Department of Pediatrics, Division of Adolescent and Young Adult Health, Vanderbilt University Medical Center, Nashville, Tennessee, USA

REBECCA L. FIX, PhD
Assistant Professor, Department of Mental Health, Johns Hopkins Bloomberg School of Public Health, Baltimore, Maryland, USA

ELIZABETH GETZOFF TESTA, PhD
Senior Psychologist, Director of Psychology Services and Research for the Center of Pediatric Weight Management and Healthy Living, Department of Psychology and Neuropsychology, Mt Washington Pediatric Hospital, Baltimore, Maryland, USA

KENNETH R. GINSBURG, MD, MSEd
Attending Pediatrician, Adolescent Medicine Specialist, Craig Dalsimer Division of Adolescent Medicine, Children's Hospital of Philadelphia, Professor, Department of Pediatrics, University of Pennsylvania Perelman School of Medicine, Founder and Program Director, Center for Parent and Teen Communication, Philadelphia, Pennsylvania, USA

CHRISTOPHER J. HAMMOND, MD, PhD
Assistant Professor, Department of Psychiatry, Division of Child and Adolescent Psychiatry, Division of Adolescent and Young Adult Medicine, Johns Hopkins University School of Medicine, Johns Hopkins Bayview Medical Center, Baltimore, Maryland, USA

SYDNEY M. HARTMAN-MUNICK, MD
Assistant Professor of Pediatrics, University of Massachusetts Memorial Children's Medical Center, UMass Chan Medical School, Worcester, Massachusetts, USA

SARAH HOLLIDAY, AGPCNP-BC, WHNP-BC
Advanced Nurse Practitioner, Division of Adolescent and Young Adult Health, Department of Pediatrics, Vanderbilt University Medical Center, Nashville, Tennessee, USA

NAT KENDALL-TAYLOR, PhD
Chief Executive Officer, FrameWorks Institute, Washington, DC, USA

BRUCE LEEWIWATANAKUL, DO
Resident, Department of Child and Adolescent Psychiatry and Behavioral Sciences, Perelman School of Medicine at the University of Pennsylvania, Children's Hospital of Philadelphia, Philadelphia, Pennsylvania, USA

JASON LEWIS, PhD
Assistant Professor of Clinical Psychiatry, Department of Child and Adolescent Psychiatry and Behavioral Sciences, The Children's Hospital of Philadelphia, University of Pennsylvania Perelman School of Medicine, Philadelphia, Pennsylvania, USA

MEREDITHE McNAMARA, MD, MSc
Assistant Professor of Pediatrics, Yale School of Medicine, New Haven, Connecticut, USA

IZABELA MILANIAK, PhD
Assistant Professor of Clinical Psychiatry, Perelman School of Medicine at the University of Pennsylvania, Department of Child and Adolescent Psychiatry and Behavioral Sciences, The Children's Hospital of Philadelphia, Philadelphia, Pennsylvania, USA

ELIZABETH MILLER, MD, PhD
Professor of Pediatrics, Public Health, and Clinical and Translational Science, Division of Adolescent and Young Adult Medicine, University of Pittsburgh School of Medicine, UPMC Children's Hospital of Pittsburgh, Pittsburgh, Pennsylvania, USA

STEVE NORTH, MD, MPH
Founder and Medical Director, Center for Rural Health Innovation, Spruce Pine, North Carolina, USA

RYAN H. PASTERNAK, MD, MPH
Professor of Pediatrics, University of Missouri-Kansas City School of Medicine, Louisiana State University School of Medicine, Children's Hospital New Orleans, New Orleans, Louisiana, USA

ANNE POWELL, MD
Assistant Professor of Pediatrics, University of Massachusetts Memorial Children's Medical Center, UMass Chan Medical School, Worcester, Massachusetts, USA

MAYA I. RAGAVAN, MD, MPH, MS
Assistant Professor of Pediatrics, Public Health, and Clinical and Translational Science, Division of General Academic Pediatrics, University of Pittsburgh School of Medicine, UPMC Children's Hospital of Pittsburgh, Pittsburgh, Pennsylvania, USA

PETER C. ROWE, MD
Professor, Department of Pediatrics, Division of Adolescent and Young Adult Medicine, Johns Hopkins School of Medicine, Baltimore, Maryland, USA

STEPHEN L. SOFFER, PhD
Professor of Clinical Psychiatry, Department of Child and Adolescent Psychiatry and Behavioral Sciences, The Children's Hospital of Philadelphia, University of Pennsylvania Perelman School of Medicine, Philadelphia, Pennsylvania, USA

ANNEMARIE McCARTNEY SWAMY, MD, PhD, FAAP, DABOM
Assistant Professor, Adolescent Medicine, Department of Pediatrics, West Virginia University, Charleston Area Medical Center, Charleston, West Virginia, USA

IDIA BINITIE THURSTON, PhD
Professor, Departments of Health Sciences and Applied Psychology, Associate Director, Institute for Health Equity and Social Justice, Affiliate Professor of Africana Studies, Northeastern University, Boston, Massachusetts, USA

KATHRYN VAN ECK, PhD
Assistant Professor of Psychiatry and Behavioral Sciences, Department of Pediatrics, Division of Adolescent and Young Adult Medicine, Johns Hopkins University School of Medicine, Kennedy Krieger Institute, Baltimore, Maryland USA

Contents

The coronavirus disease 2019 pandemic was a public health emergency that impacted adolescents across the United States and disproportionately affected youth experiencing marginalization due to less access to resources and supports. This study reviews the increases in intimate partner and youth violence during the pandemic, mechanisms contributing to these increases, and the overarching health impacts on adolescents. Pediatric health professionals have a vital role to play in implementing healing-centered practices and prevention efforts that mitigate impacts of trauma and violence and that support youth and families in pathways to healing and recovery.

Prior to COVID-19, there were already increasing rates of youth with mental health concerns, including an increase in youth presenting to medical emergency departments (EDs) with mental health chief complaints and limited access to treatment. This trend worsened during the pandemic, and rates of youth presenting to medical EDs with suicidal ideation and self-harm increased 50% from 2019 to 2022. This resulted in a "boarding" crisis, in part, due to a lack of inpatient psychiatric hospitalization beds, and many youth were left without access to adequate treatment. Additional study of innovations in health care delivery will be paramount in meeting this need.

Rates of clinical anxiety have increased during COVID and post-quarantine in youth, with older adolescent girls and youth with minorized racial, gender, and sexuality identities most vulnerable. Given that increased anxiety to a threatening/uncertain environment is adaptive, it is important to conceptualize anxiety from a balanced perspective, evaluating its functionality. For adolescents continuing to struggle with re-integration into their social environments and school avoidance, an exposure framework is necessary to

safety net resources, have politically targeted identities, are geopolitically displaced, and/or are racially or ethnically marginalized. A rapid change in social safety net policies has impacts that reverberate throughout interrelated domains of AYA health, especially for vulnerable AYAs. The authors analyze policy-related changes in mental health, climate change, and bodily autonomy to offer a paradigm for an equitable path forward.

Idia Binitie Thurston, Rebecca L. Fix, and Elizabeth Getzoff Testa

Anti-Black racism, heterosexism, and transphobia are significant public health concerns contributing to poor adolescent health outcomes. The authors introduce the health-equity adapted STYLE framework to increase knowledge and awareness of Black and lesbian, gay, bisexual, transgender, non-binary, queer, questioning, asexual, or intersex (LGBTQ) + intersectionality. Guided by case examples, the authors identify key strategies to promote anti-racist, anti-heterosexist, and anti-transphobic practices. Utilization of this framework by adolescent health providers could promote the health and well-being of Black and LGBTQ + adolescents.

PROGRAM OBJECTIVE

The goal of the *Pediatric Clinics of North America* is to keep practicing physicians and residents up to date with current clinical practice in pediatrics by providing timely articles reviewing the state-of-the-art in patient care.

TARGET AUDIENCE

All practicing pediatricians, physicians, and healthcare professionals who provide patient care to pediatric patients.

LEARNING OBJECTIVES

Upon completion of this activity, participants will be able to:

1. Review prevention and intervention strategies implemented to support youth exposed to violence post-pandemic.
2. Discuss the impact of COVID-19 on adolescent anxiety and eating disorders (EDs).
3. Recognize substance use and substance use disorders are major public health issues associated with significant societal costs.

ACCREDITATIONS

Physician Credit

The Elsevier Office of Continuing Medical Education (EOCME) is accredited by the Accreditation Council for Continuing Medical Education (ACCME) to provide continuing medical education for physicians.

The EOCME designates this journal-based activity for a maximum of 13 *AMA PRA Category 1 Credit*(s)™. Physicians should claim only the credit commensurate with the extent of their participation in the activity.

All other healthcare professionals requesting continuing education credit for this journal-based activity will be issued a certificate of participation.

ABP Maintenance of Certification Credit

Successful completion of this CME activity, which includes participation in the activity and individual assessment of and feedback to the learner, enables the learner to earn up to 13 MOC points in the American Board of Pediatrics' (ABP) Maintenance of Certification (MOC) program. It is the CME activity provider's responsibility to submit learner completion information to ACCME for the purpose of granting ABP MOC credit.

DISCLOSURE OF CONFLICTS OF INTEREST

The EOCME assesses conflict of interest with its instructors, faculty, planners, and other individuals who are in a position to control the content of CME activities. All relevant conflicts of interest that are identified are thoroughly vetted by EOCME for fair balance, scientific objectivity, and patient care recommendations. EOCME is committed to providing its learners with CME activities that promote improvements or quality in healthcare and not a specific proprietary business or a commercial interest.

The planning committee, staff, authors, and editors listed below have identified no financial relationships or relationships to products or devices they or their spouse/life partner have with commercial interest related to the content of this CME activity:

Hoover Adger, MD, MPH, MBA; Suzanne Allen, MSN, CPNP; Renata Arrington-Sanders, MD, MPH, ScM; Sarah H. Arshad, MD; Alba Azola, MD; Jesse Barondeau, MD; Tami D. Benton, MD; Debra Braun-Courville, MD; Merrian J. Brooks, DO, MS; Camille A. Broussard, MD, MPH; Joanna Brown, MD, MPH; Tina L. Cheng, MD, MPH; Elvira Chiccarelli, MD; Jeylan Close, MD; LaKeshia N. Craig, MD; Alison Culyba, MD, PhD, MPH; Stephanie Davidson, MD; Neerav Desai, MD; Errol L. Fields, MD, PhD, MPH; Rebecca L. Fix, PhD; Kenneth R. Ginsburg, MD, MSEd; Christopher J. Hammond, MD, PhD; Sydney M. Hartman-Munick, MD; Sarah Holliday, AGPCNP-BC, WHNP-BC; Shyamala Kavikumaran; Holland Kerry; Nat Kendall-Taylor, PhD; Bruce Leewiwatanakul, DO; Jason Lewis, PhD; Michelle Littlejohn; Meredithe McNamara, MD, MSc; Izabela Milaniak, PhD; Elizabeth Miller, MD, PhD; Saswoti Nath; Steve North, MD, MPH; Ryan H. Pasternak, MD, MPH; Anne Powell, MD; Maya I. Ragavan, MD, MPH, MS; Peter C. Rowe, MD; Stephen L. Soffer, PhD; Annemarie McCartney Swamy, MD, PhD; Elizabeth Getzoff Testa, PhD; Idia Binitie Thurston, PhD; Kathryn Van Eck, PhD

UNAPPROVED/OFF-LABEL USE DISCLOSURE

The EOCME requires CME faculty to disclose to the participants:

1. When products or procedures being discussed are off-label, unlabelled, experimental, and/or investigational (not US Food and Drug Administration [FDA] approved); and
2. Any limitations on the information presented, such as data that are preliminary or that represent ongoing research, interim analyses, and/or unsupported opinions. Faculty may discuss information about pharmaceutical agents that is outside of FDA-approved labelling. This information is intended solely for CME and is not intended to promote off-label use of these medications. If you have any questions, contact the medical affairs department of the manufacturer for the most recent prescribing information.

TO ENROLL
To enroll in the *Pediatric Clinics of North America* Continuing Medical Education program, call customer service at 1-800-654-2452 or sign up online at http://www.theclinics.com/home/cme. The CME program is available to subscribers for an additional annual fee of USD 313.00.

METHOD OF PARTICIPATION
In order to claim credit, participants must complete the following:
1. Complete enrolment as indicated above.
2. Read the activity.
3. Complete the CME Test and Evaluation. Participants must achieve a score of 70% on the test. All CME Tests and Evaluations must be completed online.

In order to claim MOC points, participants must complete the following:
1. Complete steps listed above for claiming CME credit
2. Provide your specialty board ID#, birth date (MM/DD), and attestation.
3. Online MOC submission is only available for the American Board of pediatrics' (ABP) Maintenance of Certification (MOC) program

CME INQUIRIES/SPECIAL NEEDS
For all CME inquiries or special needs, please contact elsevierCME@elsevier.com.

PEDIATRIC CLINICS OF NORTH AMERICA

Foreword
The Promise of Adolescence and Young Adulthood

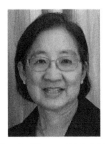

Tina L. Cheng, MD, MPH
Consulting Editor

It is a privilege to work with adolescents and young adults. I love to hear their perspectives on the world and their future. They often have a fresh outlook unencumbered by some of the biases and preconceptions that can set in with age. They are digital natives that effortlessly navigate technology and will shape the future of innovation and change.

While we collectively have experienced the trauma of a pandemic, young people have suffered but have also demonstrated great strength. This issue focuses on the impact of the pandemic on adolescents and young adults and supplements the recent National Academy of Science, Engineering, and Medicine[1] report on "Addressing the Long-Term Impact of the COVID 19 Pandemic on Children and Families." Both document the lasting adverse effects on the social, emotional, behavioral, education, mental, and physical health and well-being of children, adolescents, and young adults. Low-income families and those identifying as Black, Latino, and Native American have disproportionately borne the brunt of the negative effects.

The pandemic has worsened the "diseases of despair" (suicide, homicide, substance use), which have contributed to increased US mortality among adults as well as our young. It is more important now than ever to support young people today

Pediatr Clin N Am 71 (2024) xv–xvi
https://doi.org/10.1016/j.pcl.2024.05.006
0031-3955/24/© 2024 Published by Elsevier Inc.

pediatric.theclinics.com

and listen to and learn from their voices in addressing the challenges they face and in creating the future.

Tina L. Cheng, MD, MPH
Cincinnati Children's Hospital Medical Center
University of Cincinnati
Cincinnati Children's Research Foundation
3333 Burnet Avenue, MLC 3016
Cincinnati, OH 45229-3026, USA

E-mail address:
Tina.cheng@cchmc.org

REFERENCE

1. National Academies of Sciences, Engineering, and Medicine. 2023. Addressing the Long-Term Effects of the COVID-19 Pandemic on Children and Families. The National Academies Press; Washington, DC. Available at: https://doi.org/10. 17226/26809. Accessed May 1, 2024.

Preface

Navigating Adolescence: Pre-COVID-19 and Post-COVID-19 Pandemic

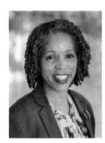
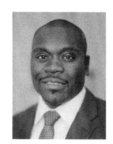

Renata Arrington-Sanders, MD, MPH, ScM   Errol L. Fields, MD, PhD, MPH
Editors

The COVID-19 pandemic disrupted the lives of adolescents globally due to social isolation; disruption of typical environments, supports and routines; loss of autonomy; and limited access to health care services. Youth simultaneously experienced discrimination, housing instability, structural racism, and other social inequities that further limited access to resources and supports important for adolescent health and well-being. This series of articles in this issue of *Pediatric Clinics of North America* is a review of the impact of COVID-19 on adolescent health, with a particular focus on post-acute sequelae of SARS-CoV-2; the increased burden of mental and behavioral health problems, exposure to violence, obesity, and other health outcomes experienced by youth after the pandemic; and the role of larger societal and structural factors (eg, policy, racism, heterosexism/transphobia) on health. This series also includes articles highlighting the resilience and innovation of adolescents and providers in the face of this adversity. Youth learned to use technology to maintain school engagement and addressed social isolation through healthy interactions with social media. Providers expanded access to clinical care through telehealth services and strategies to address structural and other barriers to adolescent health and well-being. To move forward and help youth heal from the COVID-19 pandemic, strengths-based strategies are needed to leverage youth strengths and promote different messaging that promote well-being and positive youth development. Key points and recommendations are provided for providers when addressing the needs of youth after the pandemic.

DISCLOSURE

The authors have no conflicts of interest to disclose.

Pediatr Clin N Am 71 (2024) xvii–xviii
https://doi.org/10.1016/j.pcl.2024.05.007
0031-3955/24/© 2024 Published by Elsevier Inc.

pediatric.theclinics.com

FUNDING

Dr R. Arrington-Sanders is funded by the National Institute of Health (1R01DA043089, 1R01DA059022) and receives royalties for serving as a section editor for UpToDate, Wolters Kluwer. Dr E.L. Fields is funded by the National Institutes of Health (R21MH129186-01A1).

Renata Arrington-Sanders, MD, MPH, ScM
Chief, Craig-Dalsimer Division of Adolescent Medicine
Professor of Pediatrics and Medicine
Orton Jackson Endowed Chair in Adolescent Medicine
Perelman School of Medicine, University of Pennsylvania
The Children's Hospital of Philadelphia
3501 Civic Center Boulevard
HUB, 14th Floor. Office #14581
Philadelphia, PA 19104, USA

Errol L. Fields, MD, PhD, MPH
Division of Adolescent/Young Adult Medicine
Johns Hopkins School of Medicine
200 North Wolfe Street
Room 2027
Baltimore, MD 21218, USA

E-mail addresses:
sandersr2@chop.edu (R. Arrington-Sanders)
Errol.Fields@jhmi.edu (E.L. Fields)

Supporting Youth Exposed to Violence in the Post-Pandemic

Prevention and Intervention Strategies

Alison Culyba, MD, PhD, MPH[a,b,1], Maya I. Ragavan, MD, MPH, MS[b,c,1],
Elizabeth Miller, MD, PhD[a,b,*]

KEYWORDS

- Adolescent health • Trauma • Intimate partner violence
- Adolescent relationship abuse • Youth violence • Gun violence • Dating abuse
- Health equity

KEY POINTS

- Exposure to trauma and violence is pervasive, especially youth experiencing marginalization and oppression.
- Youth already experiencing or at risk for exposure to trauma and violence were made even more vulnerable to violence exposure during the coronavirus disease 2019 pandemic.
- Provision of confidential, accessible, and affirming adolescent health services is essential during the early phases of a public health emergency (PHE) and should be maintained throughout recovery phases.
- Advocacy for youth in communities with limited access to Internet, computers, and cell phones are critical to reduce inequities in health care delivery.
- Given the multiple overlapping forms of trauma and violence that youth experience and potential barriers to disclosure, health professionals should receive training on how to offer resources and support to all patients and how to discuss options for safety and healing during the course of PHE.

---

[a] Division of Adolescent and Young Adult Medicine, Pediatrics, University of Pittsburgh School of Medicine, 120 Lytton Avenue, Pittsburgh, PA 15213, USA; [b] UPMC Children's Hospital of Pittsburgh, 4401 Penn Avenue, Pittsburgh, PA 15224, USA; [c] Division of General Academic Pediatrics, Pediatrics, University of Pittsburgh School of Medicine, 3414 5th Avenue, Pittsburgh, PA 15213, USA
[1] Denotes co-first authors.
* Corresponding author. University Center, 120 Lytton Avenue, Suite 302, Pittsburgh, PA 15213.
E-mail address: elizabeth.miller@chp.edu

Pediatr Clin N Am 71 (2024) 567–581
https://doi.org/10.1016/j.pcl.2024.04.001   pediatric.theclinics.com

INTRODUCTION

The coronavirus disease (COVID-19) pandemic (henceforth, pandemic) was a massive public health emergency (PHE) that impacted adolescents across the United States. Youth experiencing marginalization, including youth experiencing discrimination, housing instability, system involvement, immigration and language inequities, and other structural and systemic inequities, had far less access to resources and supports and bore a disproportionate burden of the pandemic on their health, academic, and social outcomes. This study reviews the rise of intimate partner and youth violence during the pandemic, identifies mechanisms contributing to both the increase in violence and the severity of violence exposure, and outlines the overarching health impacts on adolescents. We underscore the critical role for pediatric health professionals in offering research-informed, healing-centered practices to mitigate impacts of trauma and violence on children, youth, and families, and specific recommendations on how to support youth and families in pathways to healing and recovery.

PREPANDEMIC EPIDEMIOLOGY AND HEALTH IMPACTS

Even prior to the pandemic, exposure to adolescent relationship abuse (ARA), parental or caregiver intimate partner violence (IPV), and youth violence were already at epidemic proportions with significant impacts on adolescent health. In a national online survey, over two-thirds (69%) of 12 to 18 years olds who have ever dated reported ever experiencing physical, psychological, or sexual ARA.[1] Emerging literature also highlights the extent to which young people in abusive relationships, especially young people experiencing marginalization, also experience economic abuse, specifically interference with getting an education, disruptions with employment, and financial interference.[2,3] One in 4 adolescents report having been exposed to IPV in their families during their lifetime[4]; the lifetime prevalence is even higher among marginalized youth (44% in one study).[5] Data from the Centers for Disease Control and Prevention (CDC) showed an increase in sexual violence by 18% in the past decade,[6] and Healthy People 2030 data note that the prevalence of ARA is increasing.[7]

Youth and community violence are also pervasive. In a national high school-based survey in 2019, 22% of youth reported being in a physical fight and 7% reported being threatened or injured with a weapon at school in the past year.[8] Homicide, the most severe consequence of interpersonal violence, is the second leading cause of death among US youth aged 12 to 24 years and the leading cause of death among Black youth.[9–12] In the United States in 2018, 4733 adolescent and young adults (AYAs) died by homicide and over 420,000 youth received care for nonfatal assault injuries in emergency room settings. Firearm violence is also tightly linked to ARA: in one study, 14% of IPV-related homicides perpetrated by firearms were in the context of adolescent intimate relationships.[13]

ARA, caregiver IPV, and youth violence have profound impacts on health. Youth violence is associated with negative health and well-being outcomes across the life course, increasing the risk for behavioral and mental health difficulties and impacting perceived and actual safety, participation in community events, and school attendance.[14–17] ARA and exposure to caregiver IPV is associated with increased mental health symptoms, worse academic performance, substance and alcohol use, and increased reports of violence in subsequent relationships.[18–20] Leveraging strengths-based solutions is critical to prevent violence and support survivors.

EPIDEMIOLOGY OF YOUTH VIOLENCE DURING THE CORONAVIRUS DISEASE 2019 PANDEMIC

Studies have consistently found increases in prevalence and severity of IPV during PHEs and natural disasters.[21] The overall challenges with access to resources and supports that are disrupted for everyone when such disasters occur, are compounded for survivors of IPV and their children who have unique safety needs.[22,23] Additionally, the structural barriers emerging during PHEs make connection to routine supports and recovery more challenging, increasing likelihood of increased severity of IPV when PHEs occur. Among adolescents, nationally representative data from the Adolescent Behavior and Experiences Survey (conducted from January to June 2021 with over 7000 respondents) found that youth also had high levels of exposure to interpersonal violence. For example, among female-identified respondents, one in 12 (8%) experienced nondating sexual violence, 12.5% experienced sexual dating violence, and 7.7% experienced physical dating violence.[24] Anecdotally, domestic violence and crisis helplines reported increased volume of calls from youth experiencing relationship abuse. Additionally, studies have demonstrated an increase in the frequency and severity of adult IPV during the pandemic.[25,26]

Similar to increases in exposure to IPV and ARA, the number of youth experiencing assault injury increased during the pandemic and has remained elevated even as the pandemic ended. A recent review summarized the increases in violent injuries among children within the 1 year period after initiation of stay-at-home orders, primarily driven by increases in firearm injuries with the reopening of social spaces after lockdowns ended.[27] In 2020, firearm injuries became the leading cause of death for all children in the United States. Similar to overall trends, from 2018 to 2021, there was a 42% increase in the pediatric firearm death rate, with worsening disparities by race and neighborhood poverty.[28] From 2020 to 2021, Black children experienced a 12% increase in firearm homicides and multiracial youth experienced a 13% increase, while rates among white, Asian American and American Indian/Alaska Native youth remained stable to slightly increased.[28] A recent analysis using data from 40 children's hospitals demonstrated that firearm assault-related injuries increased disproportionately among youth residing in neighborhoods with concentrated disadvantage comparing prepandemic (January 2019–March 15, 2020) to during pandemic (March 16, 2020–December 2020) data.[29]

Despite the profound impact of PHEs on IPV, ARA, and community violence, to-date local and national emergency preparedness planning processes have not routinely addressed the needs of youth experiencing violence including how to provide essential health care and services in addition to ensuring safety. This lack of attention to the needs of IPV survivors during PHEs prompted the commissioning of a national report on recommendations regarding essential preventive and primary health care services related to IPV during PHEs, using an all-hazards approach, which is inclusive of natural and man-made disasters in addition to pandemics.[30] Similar to IPV, little guidance exists within emergency preparedness planning for PHEs on supports needed for youth who are made vulnerable to firearm violence exposure, particularly during these profound disruptions in social supports and service provision including with school, after-school program, shelter, and residential facility closures.

UNIQUE CHALLENGES FOR VIOLENCE-EXPOSED YOUTH DURING THE PANDEMIC, PARTICULARLY THOSE WITH MARGINALIZED IDENTITIES

Violence-exposed youth, particularly those with marginalized (or multiply marginalized) identities, faced numerous challenges during the pandemic due to intersecting structural inequities rooted in racism, concentrated poverty, digital inequities, anti-lesbian, gay, bisexual, transgender, queer, plus (LGBTQ+) policies, among others. Minoritized youth living in neighborhoods with concentrated disadvantage bear a disproportionate burden of witnessing and directly experiencing violence, which occurred even before the pandemic.[11,31–33] Minoritized youth also face barriers in accessing life-affirming resources and may experience coercive control related to their marginalized identity (eg, a gender diverse young person threatened to be "outed" by a partner or not safe living with their parents or adult caregivers). These challenges are compounded for young people with multiple marginalized identities, such as Black, Indigenous, and other People of Color (BIPOC) transgender young people. The isolation, closure of affirming and safe spaces, and anxiety during the pandemic added to the pre-existing inequities experienced by marginalized young people.

Further, the pandemic co-occurred with an international reckoning around centuries of structural racism fueled by the murder of people of African descent both within the United States and across myriad nations. This included a renewed focus on how over-policing, overrepresentation in the criminal-legal system, housing inequities including redlining, discriminatory discipline in schools, and unjust workplace practices increase risks for violence for BIPOC youth. A 2022 United Nations Report outlined international initiatives designed to address manifestations of systemic racism and noted that while progress had been made, programs overall failed to demonstrate long-overdue transformative change.[34] Particularly in the United States, this critical examination of systemic racism occurred contemporaneously with implementation of state and federal policies harmful to LGBTQ+ (including the multiple anti-trans laws in the United States and internationally) identity and expression, immigration status, and racial equity, thereby creating a nexus of oppression for BIPOC youth with multiply marginalized identities.[22]

Many youth are exposed to multiple forms of violence.[35] Youth already exposed to violence are made even more vulnerable to further exposure to trauma and violence during PHEs due to the disruptions in their already limited access to supports and resources. As an example, a young person who is experiencing violence in their home (perhaps related to their sexual or gender identity) may experience escalation of such violence during the stressors of a PHE; as this violence escalates and there are shelter-in-place orders, youth may leave their homes to find a safer place to stay, which may lead to staying with an abusive partner or sexual exploitation, food and housing insecurity, participation in survival sex (ie, exchanging sex for something of value like money, food, drugs, and a place to stay), and other vulnerabilities including physical injury and exposure to communicable diseases.[36]

The rapid uptake and now reliance on smartphones among adolescents, including at school, health care visits, and socializing, was both an important protective factor (ie, youth with phone and Internet access were able to resume school and connect with their peers much more easily) and may have contributed to increases in frequency and severity of cyber dating abuse. This broad access to multiple different forms of technology creates opportunities for abusive partners to control, stalk, and shame their partners through texts, social media, or mobile applications.[37] "Internet banging" refers to gang and group violence using social media including making threats of violence.[38] This phenomenon may be associated with the increases in youth experiencing gun violence-related assault injuries as the world began to reopen after the pandemic.

The social and physical distancing required during the COVID-19 pandemic disrupted social supports and services that help reduce violence at all socioecological levels. Especially for young people who experience marginalization and oppression from systemic racism and historical trauma, losing access to school, libraries, after-school programs, mentoring programs, employment, and other youth-serving settings profoundly disrupted critical social networks that increased their safety. The rapid closure of schools (including access to school-based mental health services), school-based health centers, clinics, and pharmacies translated to adolescents who were experiencing reproductive coercion or sexual violence losing access to safe and confidential reproductive health services. Among youth experiencing community violence, youth-serving organizations and mentoring programs were disrupted; these programs are critical lifelines that are documented to support victims and reduce reinjury.[39–42] Specifically, connections to trusted adults, peer support, and access to food and behavioral health services were all disrupted during the pandemic and slow to resume as the pandemic ended, especially in neighborhoods with concentrated disadvantage and fewer resources. Additionally, access to universal prevention programs and health education sessions that promote healthy relationships and reduce bullying and interpersonal violence were also interrupted, and similarly have been slow to rebound. This is especially true in school districts facing high levels of chronic absenteeism and persistent community violence, such that getting youth back to schools and engaged in their education remains challenging.

INNOVATIONS IN CARE FOR ADOLESCENTS DURING THE PANDEMIC THROUGH TRANSITION TO VIRTUAL SERVICES

During the pandemic, health care systems shifted rapidly to providing virtual care. Youth also transitioned to using telemedicine, and reported feeling comfortable using this technology as compared with older adults.[43] For gender diverse youth who may have limited access to affirming care, a study conducted during the pandemic found that youth were open to using telehealth to receive this specialized care.[44] Uptake of telehealth among youth has certainly increased opportunities for clinicians for provision of adolescent care (especially behavioral health). Even post-pandemic, the need for offering telehealth visits has persisted. Yet concerns about confidentiality of visits remain a major barrier for adolescent care.[45] For example, during the shelter-in-place time of the pandemic, young people reported concerns around partaking in virtual therapy due to fear that caregivers or other individuals would overhear.[36]

Youth-serving organizations and advocates identified multiple innovative ways to support young people during the pandemic.[22,23] This included making crisis lines more easily accessible via texting and confidential and anonymous chat functions, making support groups virtual, and reaching out to youth and families for "porch" conversations that maintained social distancing while dropping off food, medications, and other necessary items. A critical challenge was the lack of stable access to the Internet, data access, and phone and computer equipment (including phone chargers) needed to facilitate these relationships. Cities used municipal orders to designate frontline violence interrupters as essential health personnel, allowing violence prevention professionals to continue to deliver vital supports to youth and families in need while also protecting their health and safety through provision of personal protective equipment.[46]

APPLYING LESSONS LEARNED TO IMPROVE CLINICAL PREPAREDNESS FOR AND CARE PROVISION DURING PUBLIC HEALTH EMERGENCY

There are critical lessons learned from the pandemic and the impact on adolescent health and well-being that must be integrated into local emergency preparedness plans.[36] Even during "stable" conditions (in the absence of PHEs), adolescents, and young adults underutilize health care, often foregoing care. Places for adolescents to access confidential care are especially necessary for youth seeking sexual and reproductive health services[47] as well as prevention and care for substance use and behavioral health needs. Confidentiality has long been recognized as a core element of adolescent health care delivery, and adolescents may refuse or forego care if parental consent or notification is required.[48,49] During the pandemic, in addition to significant shifts in preventive care, the disruption to confidential clinical services was profound. For example, school-based health centers and mobile services all faced closures, interrupting care for many adolescents, including care for violence-related health concerns. The impact of such interruptions in receipt of care are still being documented. As confidentiality is foundational for providing adolescent care, part of preparing for PHEs and strengthening emergency preparedness plans is to increase access to confidential services. This includes growing school-based health centers, mobile van services, telehealth in schools, after school programs, and adolescent-friendly emergency room care. In the following sections, we outline strategies for clinicians to engage with youth and youth-serving organizations to address violence and promote well-being during PHEs and beyond.

Use of Healing-centered, Strength-based Approaches for Young People Seeking Care in Health Care Spaces

Healing-centered engagement is an approach for care provision, which prioritizes strengths and social supports. Rather than asking young people to disclose trauma or experiences, healing-centered engagement focuses on identifying important strengths, mapping social supports, and providing a nonjudgmental space that promotes wellness and thriving. Healing-centered engagement also recognizes that healing and trauma occur concurrently at the individual and collective levels. This approach also considers the healing of the youth-serving provider, understanding that trauma is pervasive and may impact providers directly or vicariously.[50,51] Healing-centered engagement happens not just at the individual provider level but also at the systems level through investment in adolescent health care infrastructure, connection to youth-serving organizations, colocated advocates, and development of policies with (rather than for) young people.[52,53] Healing-centered engagement is even more critical during a pandemic or PHE, when young people are experiencing multiple compounding stressors.

Universal Empowerment Approaches to Violence Prevention and Intervention

A key strategy for providing healing-centered approaches to youth violence prevention and intervention is the use of universal empowerment and resource provision approaches. Universal education is a research-informed strategy for offering information to *all* adolescents about teen-friendly supports and services and for helping youth access these supports. An example of universal empowerment is CUES (Confidentiality, Universal Education and Empowerment, Support), which includes provision of information around confidentiality, health information, and resources to all young people, with additional support as needed. Universal empowerment prioritizes resource provision over disclosure, which is critical, as studies have shown that young people may not share they are experiencing violence due to fear that this information will be shared without their permission.[2,54]

Key to the universal empowerment approach is implementation of scripts for clinicians to provide exact language they can use to engage young people through nonjudgmental, healing-centered approaches.[36] Additionally, through this approach, all young people are provided important community resources, which, even if not helpful for them, may be helpful for a friend or family member. In that way, information can be disseminated through networks. This approach has been tested within the context of ARA and reproductive coercion and has been shown to be effective in improving connection to resources, self-efficacy in using harm reduction strategies, and, for adolescents experiencing ARA at baseline, decreasing ARA.[55–57] This approach is also now recommended by the American Academy of Pediatrics in supporting caregivers experiencing IPV and their children.[19] Universal education is a key strategy that can be marshalled during PHEs to ensure that youth are informed about where and how to connect to support.[36] Universal education, unlike screening, is also safe to conduct through telemedicine as it does not ask young people to disclose, but rather provides needed resources. Therefore, we recommend universal education and empowerment over screening or other specific disclosure-driven strategies. **Table 1** includes sample scripts that can be used to facilitate a universal empowerment approach around violence prevention.

During preventive and acute care visits, adolescents should be asked if they have a safe, supportive adult with whom they can connect and talk. Adolescents who share that they do not have a supportive adult, or those for whom access to a supportive adult is limited due to their working several jobs or incarceration, should be offered options to connect to a youth mentor. Advocates and community violence prevention specialists identified multiple strategies for connecting with youth during the pandemic via phone, texts, video conferencing, and other virtual platforms, strategies that can be enhanced and amplified during recovery phases. Enabling and maintaining such caring connections requires access to stable sources of Internet, data access, and phone and computer equipment to sustain such adult–youth connections.

Confidentiality with Telemedicine

Unlike in-person visits, telehealth visits are neither truly private nor confidential. Clinicians cannot be guaranteed during virtual visits that there is not someone else in the room listening and cannot confirm whether adolescents feel safe speaking confidentially. Clinicians should consider and prioritize confidentiality during all parts of a visit, from scheduling to documenting. This is particularly salient during PHEs when health systems may preferentially schedule telemedicine visits. Schedulers should routinely ask when setting up virtual visits about whether the adolescent has a comfortable and private place to do the clinical encounter. If parents of caregivers are present, clinicians should request to speak alone with the adolescent, aligned with best practices during in-person visits (even while remembering that the parent/caregiver may still be in the room, simply off camera). Clinicians should consider using the private chat function during a virtual visit to assess how safe the young person feels speaking privately (although an adolescent's phone or computer may be being monitored and conversations may be being recorded).

If an adolescent does not feel safe talking during a virtual visit, providers may consider using the chat function, as long as the adolescent's phone or computer is not being monitored and conversations are not being saved. Additionally, although conducting visits virtually is safer for physical distancing, AYAs should be given a choice about completing a visit virtually or in-person. For some AYAs, health care centers may be one of the only available safe places.

Universal education can be provided by having links within the "virtual waiting room" or via the chat function during a telehealth encounter.

Should a youth disclose information about being unsafe or at risk for harm, providers should be prepared to link them to victim services agencies (using 3 way calling). If there is concern for abuse or neglect and child protective services need to be involved, clinicians are encouraged to also do 3 way calling with the young person and the representative from child welfare to discuss the situation and the young person's safety together.

Table 1 Scripts for universal education and response to violence disclosure	
Confidentiality	*I respect your privacy and it is important that you know that we discuss here is confidential. Sometimes, there may be a young person who tells me that someone has hurt them, that they are thinking about hurting themselves, or I have serious concerns about their safety, then I need to ask for help from others to keep that young person safe. What questions do you have for me about that?* A provider can signal to a young person that they do not have to disclose their story to receive support: *I know that many young people I take care of lead complicated lives. I want you to know that your story is your own. You do not have to tell me anything for me to be a support for you and to offer you information and resources. You can also tell me about a friend that you are worried about, and I am happy to share with you what we could do to help support that friend.*
Universal education	*So many of my patients have shared with me about being in unhealthy or complicated relationships, so I make sure to always share some helpful resource information to all young people, in case they ever need it to help a friend or for themselves. Young people can use these resources without using their name. Please know that if this is ever a part of your story that you would like to share with me, I am here to listen.*
Validating disclosure	*Thank you for sharing that with me. It takes so much courage to talk about this. I want to make sure you hear that no one deserves to be treated like that and it is not your fault.* *Thank you for sharing this part of your story. I hear you saying that this relationship is complicated.*
Connection to resources and to advocates	*You tell me what would be most helpful to you. I can share some information about resources that other young people in relationships like this have found helpful. I can also simply listen.* *I work really closely with some experts who know a lot about navigating complicated relationships and who have helped other young people in similar situations. They can talk to you while you are here today to share about resources that can be helpful for you, or I can give you their contact information for later.* *You can even use the phone here in my office, so it does not show up on your cell phone.* *Would you be interested in calling the [advocacy partner] together?*
Mandatory reporting	*Earlier in our visit, you may remember that I talked about times that I might need to get help from others to keep young people safe. This is one of those times—based on what you shared, I am really concerned for your safety and want to make sure you have the resources you need to stay safe. Let us talk about what this will look like and how you might want to be involved in this process.*
Connection to a trusted adult	*This is a hard situation for you. I want to make sure that you have someone you can talk to after your visit today. Who is an adult in your life that could help support you?*
	(continued on next page)

Table 1
(continued)
If the trusted adult is present: *If you would like, I can help you talk with them today. We can tell them together, or I can talk to them separately from you first then we can all talk about it together. What might be most supportive for you?*   If the trusted adult is not present: *When might be a good time to talk to them? How would you want to bring this up with them?*

Adapted from Refs.[20,36,59,60]

Collaborating with Youth-serving Community-based Agencies

While universal empowerment does not prioritize disclosure, disclosures may happen especially if the young person feels safe and secure in sharing. Key to supporting young people is listening and understanding their priorities and strengths, rather than proscriptively providing advice. Essential health and social services for adolescents include many community partners beyond the walls of health centers who can provide additional supports for young people. Having formal partnership agreements with health centers and inclusion of youth-serving organizations in integrated care plans for youth are part of ensuring less disruption of social supports and access to services and resources during PHEs and in the recovery phases. Clinicians should also focus on developing partnerships with youth-serving organizations and schools to create an ecosystem of support for children, youth, and families. Developing strong, bidirectional, and equitable partnerships outside of public health emergencies is essential, as building these de novo during a crisis is incredibly challenging. National and local infrastructure is needed to support strategic planning for how to continue to utilize these partnerships during PHEs to best serve youth and families disproportionately impacted by violence.

The Empowering Teens to Thrive (ET3) hospital-based violence intervention program and community-based mentorship program support youth injured or impacted by community violence and their families in Allegheny County, PA. Grounded in healing-centered approaches, ET3 is strategically embedded within our Center for Adolescent and Young Adult Health (CAYAH), an integrated medical and behavioral health services outpatient clinic. We provide medical follow-up, mental health support, care coordination, intensive case management, and link youth with community-based services through warm referrals (eg, housing, food assistance, and legal services). We work in collaboration with the Allegheny County Department of Human Services and the Allegheny County Health Department Office of Violence Prevention, synergizing our ET3 services with the ecosystem of school and community-based violence prevention initiatives within Allegheny County. Together, we foster a continuum of prevention and intervention services for youth and families.

Physical distancing measures necessary to manage the COVID-19 pandemic required us to transition services to virtual platforms throughout most of 2020. We were able to quickly adopt telemedicine platforms for ET3 visits for medical management, case management, and linkage to services. For the ET3 mentoring program, which began during the pandemic, we conducted all hiring and mentor trainings virtually. Mentor–mentee interactions were carried out in accordance with CDC guidelines, and therefore, they occurred remotely in 2020. In the context of the pandemic, we found that many injured youth did not have the capacity to connect with community-based mentors in the immediate post-injury period, in part due to technology challenges previously highlighted. We pivoted to porch drop-offs and in-person outdoor meetups to mitigate these challenges. We also broadened our inclusion criteria for the mentorship component to include youth impacted by community violence, including those who had lost an immediate family member to gun violence. We recognized the importance of giving youth opportunities to share their stories of coping and recovery to better understand how ET3 could support teens to thrive during the pandemic and through recovery phases. ET3 mentors have deep roots in the communities they serve, and their connections with community organizations are fundamental to their ability to serve as trusted messengers in their communities during public health emergencies. As we emerge from the pandemic, many ET3 participants continue to face structural inequities that constrain their access to resources and opportunities and put them and their loved ones at risk for violence. ET3 is strategically positioned within the ecosystem of violence prevention and intervention programs in the county and working closely with youth-serving organizations to provide wrap around support.

Inclusion of Youth and Community Voice in Developing Public Health Emergency Plans

Youth-serving organizations as well as youth who have been exposed to violence have experiences from provision of and receipt of care during the pandemic, respectively, that are critical to inform emergency preparedness for PHEs. People with lived experience should be involved in discussions and trainings associated with emergency preparedness including ensuring that services are accessible and linguistically and culturally responsive. There is ample example from community partner leadership around COVID-19 vaccine access and trustworthiness, including youth involvement. As an example, the Community Vitality Collaborative is a community-academic collaboration, with community partners leading vaccine trial recruitment, implementation of community-based vaccine clinics, development of processes to prioritize vaccine access for non-English speaking communities, older adults, and communities with disabilities, and coconducting research.[58] Key to the CVC was a youth group, who developed infographics around vaccines, supported young people who lost caregivers due to the pandemic, and engaged with adult collaborators to ensure young people had access to the vaccine. Similar youth-partnered approaches are essential to uplift youth voices and agency.

Lessons Learned About Supporting Staff and Clinicians' Wellness

Supporting the mental well-being of frontline staff and clinicians is a key tenet of healing-centered engagement and should be integrated into routine practice (not solely during PHEs, and attention to wellness and staff support needs to be increased during PHEs). These strategies include (1) development of self-care plans; (2) group support sessions; and (3) flexible work schedules to accommodate caregiver responsibilities, including sick leave and paid time off. Investment in adolescent and young adult health, through equitable pay for clinicians and staff to promote retention and thriving, adequate and healing-centered clinical spaces (eg, space for colocated advocates), mobile clinics to provide care within communities, and youth collaboratives to design clinical spaces are also critical to combat moral injury experienced by youth-serving clinicians and provide the services and supports that our young people deserve.

SUMMARY

Clinicians serving young people have an urgent responsibility to collaboratively and creatively support youth exposed to or experiencing violence during PHEs such as a pandemic.

Adolescent confidential services and access to comprehensive care need to be categorized as essential health services during PHE and enhanced in the recovery phases. Violence prevention professionals should be considered essential personnel, allowing them to continue to serve youth and families during times of heightened risk of violence.

Formal partnership agreements between health centers serving adolescents and youth-serving community organizations including victim service advocates and mentoring programs are critical for growing supports and services for youth, especially young people experiencing marginalization and structural inequities.

CLINICS CARE POINTS

- Clinicians should use healing-centered approaches to support all youth, recognizing that exposure to trauma and violence impacts far too many young people, especially youth experiencing marginalization and oppression, with heightened risks during PHEs.

- Clinicians should work with health systems to ensure provision of confidential, accessible adolescent health services as essential services during PHEs to safeguard child and adolescent health.

- Providers can play an important role in advocacy for youth in communities with limited access to Internet, computers, and cellphones to promote equitable health care delivery.

- Given the multiple overlapping forms of trauma and violence that youth experience, health professionals should be prepared to offer resources and support to all patients regardless of disclosure and discuss options for safety and healing during all phases of PHEs.

- Clinicians should develop partnerships with youth-serving organizations and leverage these partnerships to support youth and families during PHEs.

DISCLOSURE

Dr E. Miller receives royalties for writing content for UpToDate, Wolters Kluwer. Drs M.I. Ragavan and A. Culyba have nothing to disclose.

REFERENCES

1. Taylor BG, Mumford EA. A national descriptive portrait of adolescent relationship abuse: results from the national survey on teen relationships and intimate violence. J Interpers Violence 2016;31(6):963–88.
2. Scott SE, Lavage DR, Risser L, et al. Economic Abuse and Help-Seeking Intentions Among Adolescents. J Interpers Violence 2024;39(1–2):107–32.
3. Scott S, Lavage DR, Acharya G, et al. Experiences of exploitation and associations with economic abuse in adolescent dating relationships: findings from a U.S. Cross-Sectional Survey. J Trauma & Dissociation 2023;24(4):489–505.
4. Hamby S, Finkelhor D, Turner H, Ormrod R. Children's Exposure to Intimate Partner Violence and Other Family Violence. Washington DC: Office of Juvenile Justice and Delinquency Prevention; 2011.
5. Ragavan MI, Culyba AJ, Shaw D, et al. Social support, exposure to parental intimate partner violence, and relationship abuse among marginalized youth. J Adolesc Health 2020;67(1):127–30.
6. Youth risk behavior survey DATA SUMMARY & TRENDS REPORT 2011-2021. Centers for Disease Control and Prevention; 2023.
7. Violence prevention - healthy people 2030 | health.gov. Available at: https://health.gov/healthypeople/objectives-and-data/browse-objectives/violence-prevention. [Accessed 5 November 2023].

8. Basile KC, Clayton HB, DeGue S, et al. Interpersonal violence victimization among high school students - youth risk behavior survey, United States, 2019. MMWR Suppl 2020;69(1):28–37.
9. Cunningham RM, Walton MA, Carter PM. The major causes of death in children and adolescents in the united states. N Engl J Med 2018;379(25):2468–75.
10. David-Ferdon C., Vivolo-Kantor A.M., Dahlberg L.L., A comprehensive technical package for the prevention of youth violence and associated risk behaviors. Report. Atlanta, GA: National Center for Injury Prevention and Control, Centers for Disease Control and Prevention, 2016. Available at: https://stacks.cdc.gov/view/cdc/43085. Accessed April 30, 2024.
11. Underwood JM, Brener N, Thornton J, et al. Youth risk behavior surveillance — United States, 2019. Centers for Disease Control and Prevention; 2020. Available at: http://www.cdc.gov/healthyyouth/data/yrbs/pdf/2019/su6901-H.pdf. [Accessed 6 June 2022].
12. Web-based Injury Statistics Query and Reporting System (WISQARS). Harvard Dataverse 2009. https://doi.org/10.7910/dvn/n8emxe.
13. Wilson RF, Xu L, Betz CJ, et al. Firearm homicides of us children precipitated by intimate partner violence: 2003-2020. Pediatrics 2023;152(6). https://doi.org/10.1542/peds.2023-063004.
14. Browning CR, Gardner M, Maimon D, et al. Collective efficacy and the contingent consequences of exposure to life-threatening violence. Dev Psychol 2014;50(7):1878–90.
15. Sumner SA, Mercy JA, Dahlberg LL, et al. Violence in the united states: status, challenges, and opportunities. JAMA 2015;314(5):478–88.
16. David-Ferdon C., Simon T.R., *Preventing Youth Violence: Opportunities for Action.* Report. Atlanta, GA: National Center for Injury Prevention and Control, Centers for Disease Control and Prevention, 2014. Available at: https://stacks.cdc.gov/view/cdc/23501. Accessed April 30, 2024.
17. Houry DE, Mercy JA. *Preventing Multiple Forms of Violence: A Strategic Vision for Connecting the Dots.* Division of Violence Prevention. Atlanta, GA: National Center for Injury Prevention and Control, Centers for Disease Control and Prevention; 2016.
18. Exner-Cortens D, Eckenrode J, Rothman E. Longitudinal associations between teen dating violence victimization and adverse health outcomes. Pediatrics 2013;131(1):71–8.
19. Thackeray J, Livingston N, Ragavan MI, et al. Intimate partner violence: role of the pediatrician. Pediatrics 2023;152(1). https://doi.org/10.1542/peds.2023-062509.
20. Ragavan MI, Barral RL, Randell KA. Addressing adolescent relationship abuse in the context of reproductive health care. Semin Reprod Med 2022;40(1–02):146–54.
21. Brabete AC, Wolfson L, Stinson J, et al. Exploring the linkages between substance use, natural disasters, pandemics, and intimate partner violence against women: a rapid review in the context of COVID-19. Sexes 2021;2(4):509–22.
22. Risser L, Berger RP, Renov V, et al. Supporting children experiencing family violence during the COVID-19 pandemic: IPV and CPS provider perspectives. Acad Pediatr 2022;22(5):842–9.
23. Ragavan MI, Risser L, Duplessis V, et al. The impact of the COVID-19 pandemic on the needs and lived experiences of intimate partner violence survivors in the United States: advocate perspectives. Violence Against Women 2022;28(12–13):3114–34.

24. Krause KH, DeGue S, Kilmer G, et al. Prevalence and correlates of non-dating sexual violence, sexual dating violence, and physical dating violence victimization among u.s. high school students during the COVID-19 pandemic: adolescent behaviors and experiences survey, United States, 2021. J Interpers Violence 2023;38(9–10):6961–84.
25. Peitzmeier SM, Fedina L, Ashwell L, et al. Increases in intimate partner violence during COVID-19: prevalence and correlates. J Interpers Violence 2022; 37(21–22):NP20482–512.
26. Kourti A, Stavridou A, Panagouli E, et al. Domestic violence during the COVID-19 pandemic: a systematic review. Trauma Violence Abuse 2023;24(2):719–45.
27. Georgeades C, Flynn-O'Brien KT. The effects of the COVID-19 pandemic on violent injuries in children: a literature review. Adv Pediatr 2023;70(1):17–44.
28. Roberts BK, Nofi CP, Cornell E, et al. Trends and disparities in firearm deaths among children. Pediatrics 2023;152(3). https://doi.org/10.1542/peds.2023-061296.
29. Haasz M, Hanson H, Pomerantz W, et al. Disparities in pediatric firearm injuries during the covid-19 pandemic: a multicenter retrospective cohort study. Oral Presentation at American Academy of Pediatrics NCE Conference 2023.
30. National Academies. Sustaining essential health care services related to intimate partner violence during public health emergencies. Available at: https://www.nationalacademies.org/our-work/sustaining-essential-health-care-services-related-to-intimate-partner-violence-during-public-health-emergencies. [Accessed 16 December 2023].
31. McDonald CC, Deatrick JA, Kassam-Adams N, et al. Community violence exposure and positive youth development in urban youth. J Community Health 2011; 36(6):925–32.
32. Finkelhor D, Turner HA, Shattuck A, et al. Prevalence of childhood exposure to violence, crime, and abuse: results from the national survey of children's exposure to violence. JAMA Pediatr 2015;169(8):746–54.
33. Hardaway CR, McLoyd VC, Wood D. Exposure to violence and socioemotional adjustment in low-income youth: an examination of protective factors. Am J Community Psychol 2012;49(1–2):112–26.
34. United Nations High Commissioner for Human Rights. Promotion and protection of the human rights and fundamental freedoms of Africans and of people of African descent against excessive use of force and other human rights violations by law enforcement officers through transformative change for racial justice and equality - report of the. United Nations High Commissioner for Human Rights; 2022. Available at: https://www.ohchr.org/en/documents/thematic-reports/ahrc5153-promotion-and-protection-human-rights-and-fundamental-freedoms. [Accessed 16 December 2023].
35. Wilkins N, Tsao B, Hertz M, et al. *Connecting the Dots: An Overview of the Links among Multiple Forms of Violence*. Atlanta, GA: National Center for Injury Prevention and Control, Centers for Disease Control and Prevention; 2014.
36. Ragavan MI, Culyba AJ, Muhammad FL, et al. Supporting adolescents and young adults exposed to or experiencing violence during the covid-19 pandemic. J Adolesc Health 2020;67(1):18–20.
37. Bansal V, Rezwan M, Iyer M, et al. A scoping review of technology-facilitated gender-based violence in low- and middle-income countries across Asia. Trauma Violence Abuse 2023;4. https://doi.org/10.1177/15248380231154614. 15248380231154614.

38. Moule RK, Pyrooz DC, Decker SH. Internet adoption and online behaviour among american street gangs. Br J Criminol 2014;54(6):1186–206.
39. Lumba-Brown A, Batek M, Choi P, et al. Mentoring pediatric victims of interpersonal violence reduces recidivism. J Interpers Violence 2020;35(21–22):4262–75.
40. Cheng TL, Haynie D, Brenner R, et al. Effectiveness of a mentor-implemented, violence prevention intervention for assault-injured youths presenting to the emergency department: results of a randomized trial. Pediatrics 2008;122(5):938–46.
41. Tolan PH, Henry DB, Schoeny MS, et al. Mentoring programs to affect delinquency and associated outcomes of youth at-risk: a comprehensive meta-analytic review. J Exp Criminol 2014;10(2):179–206.
42. Lindstrom Johnson S, Jones V, Ryan L, et al. Investigating effects of mentoring for youth with assault injuries: results of a randomized-controlled trial. Prev Sci 2022; 23(8):1414–25.
43. Evans YN, Golub S, Sequeira GM, et al. Using telemedicine to reach adolescents during the COVID-19 pandemic. J Adolesc Health 2020;67(4):469–71.
44. Sequeira GM, Kidd KM, Coulter RWS, et al. Transgender youths' perspectives on telehealth for delivery of gender-affirming care. J Adolesc Health 2021;68(6): 1207–10.
45. Rankine J, Kidd KM, Sequeira GM, et al. Adolescent perspectives on the use of telemedicine for confidential health care: an exploratory mixed-methods study. J Adolesc Health 2023;73(2):360–6.
46. City of Los Angeles. Public order under city of los angeles emergency authority. 2020. Available at: https://www.lamayor.org/sites/g/files/wph446/f/article/files/ SAFER_AT_HOME_ORDER2020.03.19.pd. [Accessed 17 December 2023].
47. Miller MK, Mollen CJ. Critical access to care: bringing contraception to adolescents in nontraditional settings. J Adolesc Health 2017;61(6):667–8.
48. Ford C, English A, Sigman G. Confidential health care for adolescents: position paper for the society for adolescent medicine. J Adolesc Health 2004;35(2): 160–7.
49. Greydanus DE, Patel DR. Consent and confidentiality in adolescent health care. Pediatr Ann 1991;20(2):80–4.
50. Ragavan MI, Miller E. Healing-centered care for intimate partner violence survivors and their children. Pediatrics 2022;149(6). https://doi.org/10.1542/peds. 2022-056980.
51. Ginwright S. The future of healing: shifting from trauma informed care to healing centered engagement. 2018. Available at: https://ginwright.medium.com/the-future-of-healing-shifting-from-trauma-informed-care-to-healing-centered-engagement-634f557ce69c. [Accessed 23 April 2021].
52. Ragavan MI, Garg A, Raphael JL. Creating healing-centered health systems by reimagining social needs screening and supports. JAMA Pediatr 2023;177(6): 555–6.
53. Ragavan MI, Murray A. Supporting intimate partner violence survivors and their children in pediatric healthcare settings. Pediatr Clin North Am 2023;70(6): 1069–86.
54. Lippy C, Jumarali SN, Nnawulezi NA, et al. The impact of mandatory reporting laws on survivors of intimate partner violence: intersectionality, help-seeking and the need for change. J Fam Violence 2020;35(3):255–67.
55. Miller E, Goldstein S, McCauley HL, Jones KA, et al. A school health center intervention for abusive adolescent relationships: a cluster RCT. Pediatrics 2015; 135(1):76–85.

56. Miller E, Tancredi DJ, Decker MR, et al. A family planning clinic-based intervention to address reproductive coercion: a cluster randomized controlled trial. Contraception 2016;94(1):58–67.
57. Miller E, Jones KA, McCauley HL, et al. Cluster randomized trial of a college health center sexual violence intervention. Am J Prev Med 2020;59(1):98–108.
58. Krakora M, Townsend T, Castillo Smyntek XA, et al. From vaccines to vitality: the progression of a community-academic collaboration. Health Promot Pract 2022; 8. https://doi.org/10.1177/15248399221137271. 15248399221137272.
59. Jarvis L, Randell KA. The health care provider's role in addressing adolescent relationship abuse. Pediatr Clin North Am 2023;70(6):1087–102.
60. Miller E. Healing-Centered Engagement: Fostering Connections Rather than Forcing Disclosures. In: Ginsburg KR, Brett Z, McClain R, editors. Reaching Teens: Strength-Based, Trauma-Sensitive, Resilience-Building Communication Strategies Rooted In Positive Youth Development. American Academic of Pediatrics; Chicago, IL, 2020. Chapter 31, p. 1-3.

Adolescent Health in the Post-Pandemic Era
Evolving Stressors, Interventions, and Prevention Strategies amid Rising Depression and Suicidality

Jeylan Close, MD[a,b,*], Sarah H. Arshad, MD[c],
Stephen L. Soffer, PhD[d], Jason Lewis, PhD[d], Tami D. Benton, MD[d]

KEYWORDS

- Adolescent • Mental health • Child and adolescent psychiatry • Depression
- COVID-19 • Suicide, suicidality, suicidal ideation

KEY POINTS

- The COVID pandemic was associated with numerous stressors for youth and a rise in mental health concerns, with increased disparities seen with certain minority youth populations. There are numerous contributing factors to the worsening mental health of youth during this period.
- In 2020, there was rise in emergency department (ED) visits for youth mental health concerns and in 2021, nearly a rise in ED visits for suspected suicide attempts, especially by teenage girls (compared to 2019). Pediatric EDs faced a boarding crisis, as there were insufficient inpatient psychiatric hospital beds available for treatment of these youth.

Continued

INTRODUCTION

In October 2021, 3 major organizations serving children—the American Academy of Pediatrics (AAP), the American Academy of Child and Adolescent Psychiatry

[a] National Clinician Scholars Program, Department of Psychiatry and Behavioral Sciences, Child & Family Mental Health & Community Psychiatry Division, Duke University School of Medicine, 710 West Main Street, Durham, NC 27701, USA; [b] Duke Margolis Center for Health Policy, Duke University, 710 West Main Street, Durham, NC 27701, USA; [c] Children's Hospital of Philadelphia, University of Pennsylvania Perelman School of Medicine and UC Irvine School of Medicine, The Hub for Clinical Collaboration, DCAPBS, Floor 12, 3500 Civic Center Boulevard, Philadelphia, PA 19104, USA; [d] Department of Child and Adolescent Psychiatry and Behavioral Sciences, Children's Hospital of Philadelphia and University of Pennsylvania Perelman School of Medicine, 4601 Market Street, 3rd Floor, Philadelphia, PA 19139, USA
* Corresponding author. Duke Margolis Center for Health Policy, Duke University, 710 West Main Street, Durham, NC 27701.
E-mail address: Jeylan.Close@Duke.edu

Pediatr Clin N Am 71 (2024) 583–600
https://doi.org/10.1016/j.pcl.2024.04.002   pediatric.theclinics.com

Continued

- The lack of care as expected—both from lack of inpatient psychiatric hospital beds but also the shutdown of in-home services and in person therapy—necessitated alternate forms of intervention and hopes for prevention.
- Promising models of increasing access to mental health services include the collaborative care model with pediatricians and school-based services.
- The US Surgeon General's 2021 report on youth mental health emphasizes the importance of focusing on ensuring access to effective mental health care, creating environments in the school, home, and community that are supportive of positive mental health, and addressing societal factors that may contribute to poor mental health outcomes.

(AACAP), and the Children's Hospital Association (CHA)—declared a national emergency in children's mental health, noting the multifold detrimental impact of the COVID-19 pandemic on children's mental health, including adversity, disruption, loss of safety and structure, and disproportionate impacts on children of color due to structural racism.[1] Many children and families found their lives dramatically altered, whether trying to work or attend school from home, becoming socially isolated from activities and communities, experiencing traumatic loss with the morbidity and mortality of family members, and overall losing any sense of normalcy or connection to previously stability and structure. From April 2020 through June 2021, more than 140,000 youth lost a parent, a guardian, or a caregiver.[2] Due to many factors, there were increasing rates of youth mental health conditions and crises, including depression, anxiety, and trauma, as well as youth with suicidal ideation.

Prior to the pandemic, there was already a notable lack of sufficient resources for pediatric mental health, including access to care as well as specific disparities faced by certain minority youth. During COVID, due to the uptick in mental health crises as well as some pandemic-related factors, there was an even greater scarcity of inpatient psychiatric hospital beds for youth, leading to a "boarding" crisis in pediatric emergency departments (EDs) and hospitals, which were ill equipped to care for these youth.[3]

EPIDEMIOLOGY AND ACCESS TO CARE
Pre-2020: Before the COVID-19 Pandemic

The youth mental health crisis was exacerbated by the events in 2020, but the picture was worsening in the years leading up to the pandemic. The national prevalence of at least one mental health disorder in a 2016 national survey of youth was estimated to be 16.5%.[4] At that time, it was estimated that about half of the children with a diagnosed mental health condition did not receive treatment from a mental health professional.[4] Engagement in care in rural communities was even worse, with about 70% of youth with an identified psychiatric disorder never receiving psychiatric treatment.[5]

From 2011 to 2015, mental health-related ED visits increased by 54% for adolescents.[6] The increase from 2011 to 2015 was especially notable in Black (53%) and Hispanic (91%) youth.[6] Another study from 2011 to 2020, found an average 8% increase in mental health-related ED visits per year for adolescents.[7] The average yearly increase for suicide-related ED visits was 23.1%, and by 2020 accounted for about 5% of all pediatric ED visits.[7]

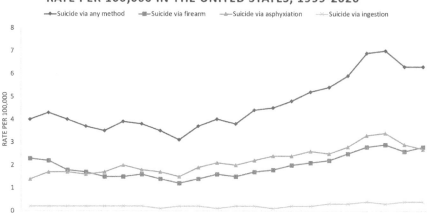

RATE PER 100,000 IN THE UNITED STATES, 1999-2020

Fig. 1. Cause of death of children aged 12 to 17 years.[8] (*Source*: Data from CDC WONDER Underlying Causes of Death were used. (does not require permission).)

Rates of youth suicide increased over the course of the 2010s (**Fig. 1**).[8] From 1999 to 2020, firearms remained the most common method of suicide for male individuals and asphyxiation remained the most common method for female individuals.[9] Of suicide attempts via ingestion from 2019 to 2022, acetaminophen and ibuprofen were the most common substances.[10]

2020 to 2021: Height of the COVID-19 Pandemic

In 2020, more than 1 in 10 youth in the United States reported that they experienced symptoms of depression that severely impacted their functioning.[11] Suicide was the second leading cause of death for children aged 10 to 14 years and the third leading cause for those aged 15 to 24 years.[12] Scarcity of specialty mental health care was exacerbated as the COVID-19 pandemic increased need and affected provider availability. Approximately 60% of youth with major depression in 2020 did not receive any care from mental health professionals.[11] For Asian youth with major depression in 2020, 78% did not receive care from a mental health specialist.[11] Access to services was especially difficult for the more than 10% of youth whose insurance did not provide coverage for mental or emotional conditions.[11]

In 2020, pediatric EDs saw a 24% increase in visits for youth mental health concerns.[13] There was specifically a rise in pediatric emergency department (ED) visits for children and adolescents facing mental health emergencies, including a nearly 51% increase in emergency room visits for suspected suicide attempts by teenage girls in early 2021, when compared with 2019.[14]

Data from the 2021 Centers for Disease Control and Prevention (CDC)'s Youth Risk Behavior Survey (YRBS) indicated that youth symptoms of depression and suicidality continued to worsen (**Fig. 2**).[15] Between 2019 and 2021, the YRBS data also indicate that Black and Hispanic youth had the steepest increases in feeling persistently sad and hopeless (**Fig. 3**).[15]

2022 to 2023: After COVID-19 Vaccine Availability

Trends for youth mental health continued to worsen through 2022 to 2023. From 2016 to 2022, ED visits for mental health concerns tripled.[16] Suicidal ideation and self-harm-related ED visits increased 50% from 2019 to 2022.[16]

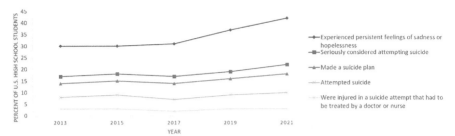

Fig. 2. CDC Youth Risk Behavior Study data on high school student mental health.[15] (*Source*: Data from the CDC Youth Risk Behavior Study (YRBS) were used (does not require permission).)

A national analysis of commercial insurance claims examined mental health-related utilization between 3 periods: (1) "baseline," March 2019 to February 2020; (2) "pandemic year 1," March 2020 to February 2021; and (3) "pandemic year 2," March 2021 to February 2022.[17] The study found that the percent of youth who had a mental health-related outpatient visit in the 30 days prior to their ED visit decreased from 78.1% to 76.3% to 72.2% over the 3 times.[17] The percent of youth who waited

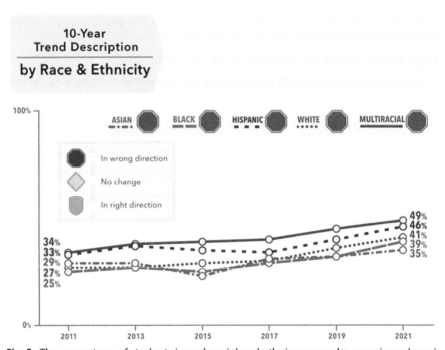

Fig. 3. The percentage of students in each racial and ethnic group who experienced persistent feelings of sadness or hopelessness from 2011 to 2021[15]. (*Source*: Figure is from the CDC Youth Risk Behavior Study (YRBS) Data Summary & Trends Report[15] (Does not require permission. Reference to the figure does not constitute endorsement or recommendation by the U.S. Government, Department of Health and Human Services, or Centers for Disease Control and Prevention. The figure is otherwise available on the agency website at CDC.gov for no charge).)

more than 2 midnights in an ED for an acute psychiatric hospitalization increased 27.1% from "baseline" to "pandemic year 1" and 76.4% from "baseline" to "pandemic year 2."[17] Combined, these data indicate that fewer youth with mental health concerns are receiving outpatient care prior to crises and there has continued to be a marked increase in extended ED stays, termed "boarding." In addition to the inadequate mental health specialist workforce, barriers exist within primary care to provide first-line mental health care.[18] The majority of pediatricians report that they feel they have had inadequate training in mental health and lack of confidence in managing mental health conditions.[18] Over the course of 2019 to 2022, ED visits for female suicidality and self-harm increased 43.6% and eating disorder diagnoses increased 120.4%,[17] but no significant increases in ED visits for male individuals of any diagnostic categories were observed.[17]

The Trevor Project's 2023 National Survey on the Mental Health of Lesbian, Gay, Bisexual, Transgender, and Queer (LGBTQ) Young People showed similar trends from CDC's 2021 YRBS data (**Fig. 4**).[15,19] About 41% of LGBTQ youth in the 2023 survey seriously considered suicide, compared to 45% in 2021.[15,19] The 2023 survey also found that about half of transgender and nonbinary youth seriously considered suicide, although a lower percentage considered suicide if they felt their school was gender-affirming.[19] The survey found that similar to pre-2020, half of youth seeking mental health care were unable to receive it.[4,19] Further, it is also known that the intersectionality of multiple minoritized identities, such as racial and gender identities, is associated with higher rates of suicidal ideation.[20]

Beyond May 2023: The End of the COVID-19 Public Health Emergency

At the time of this publication, it is too early for available data on epidemiology for mental health concerns after the end of the COVID-19 Public Health Emergency (PHE), which was declared in May 2023. With the federally declared ending of the PHE, new stressors have been introduced. Specifically, as states begin Medicaid "unwinding," or redetermination of Medicaid eligibility that was paused during the PHE, many children and adolescents may lose health insurance.[21] It is estimated that 3.8 million children and adolescents who are still eligible will lose their Medicaid coverage due to administrative issues, and subsequently will be unable to receive mental health services.[21] Additionally, the effects of systemic racism continue to be present, and laws targeting minority and LGBTQ+ youth continue to be passed in many states.[22,23] The additional stressors come as children are still dealing with the grief and isolation they experienced during the earlier phases of the pandemic.

CONTRIBUTING FACTORS TO DEPRESSION AND SUICIDAL IDEATION IN ADOLESCENTS
Structural Inequities and Racial Injustice

According to the CDC, there have been over 1 million deaths due to COVID-19 since 2020.[24] In the initial 6 months, racial and ethnic disparities in hospitalization and

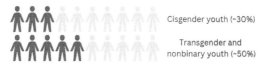

Cisgender youth (~30%)

Transgender and nonbinary youth (~50%)

Fig. 4. Percentage of LGBTQ youth who seriously considered suicide in 2023.[19] (*Source*: Data from Trevor Project's 2023 National Survey on the Mental Health LGBTQ Young People were used (does not require permission).)

mortality were clearly delineated,[25] highlighting the disproportionate impact of the pandemic on the morbidity and mortality of minorities and low income populations, and showcasing the impact of structural inequalities on social determinants of health.[26] Early in the pandemic, incidence of COVID-19 was higher in zip codes with higher minority populations[27]; this was also the time when health care systems were the least informed and prepared to treat these patients and families. Youth in these zip codes, mostly from lower income families and with minority cultural backgrounds, were also affected, not only by viral infection but also by secondary devastation as their households and communities were disproportionately destabilized and suffering. These youth were less able to rely on adults for their own support, connectedness, and to cope with their responses to stress. Caregiver losses occurred with greater rates in racial minorities, with caregiver death affecting "1 of 753 White children, 1 of 682 Asian children, 1 of 412 Hispanic children, 1 of 310 Black children, and 1 of 168 American Indian and/or Alaska Native children".[2]

In addition, in 2019 the AAP came out with a policy statement about the impact of racism on child and adolescent health, highlighting racism as a social determinant of health that has a "profound impact" on the health of youth and their families, especially diverse youth, including how exposure to chronic stress (and stress hormones) can biologically drive chronic disease.[28] The statement also reports that youth who directly experience racism sustain the most impact, but that bystanders are also negatively affected. A study of Black American adults found negative mental health outcomes associated when they were exposed to police killing of unarmed Black Americans.[29] It is important to note that Black youth are also exposed to repetitive bystander stress and ultimately trauma at witnessing (whether firsthand or later, via media or social media) incidents of racial profiling and police brutality. They were also exposed to the increasingly public murders of many Black Americans, including some youth, in the years leading up to the COVID pandemic.[30] In 2020, they faced an additional stressor with the murder of George Floyd by police officers in May 2020, caught on camera telling police officers that he could not breathe, which sparked a fierce movement to combat racial injustice. Other minority youth were also affected by racial injustice and racial targeting—there was an increase in students reporting experiencing racism, especially among Asian youth (64%) and Black and multiple race youth (55%).[31] Community leaders in Generation Z often led protests and advocacy for police reform.[32]

Social Isolation

Social isolation was experienced by all youth during the pandemic, especially with virtual school in place of in-person school attendance and the normalization of social distancing to combat the pandemic spread. Studies depict the negative impact of social isolation on youth mental health, including higher rates of anxiety and depression and emotional development.[33,34] In the Surgeon General's 2023 report on loneliness, Dr. Murthy states that the association of social disconnection with mortality is similar to smoking 15 cigarettes a day, which is higher than the association with obesity and inactivity.[34] Many youth lost the protective factor of "social connectedness" through school during the pandemic.[31] Social distancing was associated with more stress and anxiety for economically disadvantaged children.[35]

Adverse Childhood Experiences

Beyond losing social connections, youth were also exposed to greater amounts of trauma during this time, including both traumatic loss from the death of loved ones, as well as from abuse. In 2021, 55% of youth reported experiencing emotional abuse by a parent or adult in the home, 11% reported physical abuse, and 24% reported they did not have enough food to eat.[31,36] In addition, the pandemic saw an 8.1% increase in domestic violence, often affecting many households with children.[37]

Lack of Mental Health Care Access

With increasing rates of pediatric mental health problems, there has been a growing demand for services from an already under-resourced system. Unfortunately, the COVID-19 pandemic itself has had a significant negative impact on available health care resources used to target pediatric mental health, which, in turn, has also been a factor in the increasing prevalence and severity of pediatric depression and suicidal ideation. There is reduced availability across all levels of care.

It is estimated that there are only about 5 clinical child and adolescent psychologists and 14 child and adolescent psychiatrists per 100,000 youth aged under 18 years.[38,39] The majority of counties in the United States have zero child and adolescent psychologists or psychiatrists (**Fig. 5**).[38,39] Furthermore, there are no states that have a sufficient amount of recommended school-based mental health support staff, such as school counselors, social workers, and psychologists.[40] The shortages mean that children are waiting months to establish care when they are in need.[41]

At the highest level of service, there has been a decrease in the number of inpatient psychiatric beds. Many psychiatric units converted their beds to general medical units, and of those units that have remained, there have been instances of double rooms being converted to single rooms.[42] Furthermore, children and adolescents on inpatient units requiring discharge to lower levels of care, such as residential facilities or partial hospitalization programs, have had their stays on the inpatient units extended due to a lack of availability in these stepdown programs.[43] As a consequence of this bottleneck on pediatric psychiatric inpatient units, depressed children and adolescents arriving to pediatric medical EDs end up facing the sobering reality that there is often nowhere to go. The preexisting problem of "boarding," defined by the Joint Commission as the practice of holding patients in the ED for another temporary location after the decision to admit or transfer has been made,[44] has thus been exacerbated.[45] A 2022 survey of 88 United States hospitals found that 98.9% reported that their hospitals boarded children awaiting inpatient psychiatric care and 84.4% reported increased boarding during the pandemic.[46] At the same time, because of the far-reaching negative effects of the pandemic, there has been a sharp increase in visits

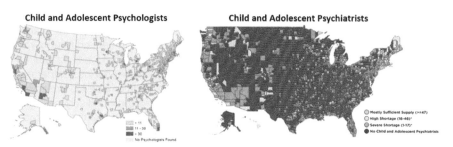

Fig. 5. Geographic distribution of child and adolescent psychologist and psychiatrist per 100k youth 18 years old or younger[38,39]. (*Source*: Figure on the left is from the University of Michigan Behavioral Health Workforce Research Center and American Psychological Association[39] (Reproduced with permission from American Psychological Association. No further reproduction or distribution is permitted.). Figure on the right is from the American Academy of Child and Adolescent Psychiatry Workforce Maps by State[39] (does not require permission).)

to EDs for mental health problems.[47] As a result, the sum impact is an increase in depressed children and adolescents presenting to EDs and few options for them once they are ready to be discharged to initiate ongoing mental health care.

COSTS AND CONSEQUENCES

Before the pandemic, the yearly national expenditure on children with mental health diagnoses was around $8.8 billion.[48] In 2016, it was estimated that 55% of all Medicaid spending for youth went to those with a mental health condition.[49] Since 2020, private insurance providers reported an estimated 186% surge in expenses for dependents diagnosed with mental health conditions, likely related to the marked rise in mental health crises and ED visits.[14,50] Increased rates of depression also have downstream costs, including lower academic performance, higher engagement in crime, and generational transmission of mental health issues.[51]

With the dearth of outpatient mental health providers, families are having to drive multiple hours to appointments and pay high prices to find care.[41] One in 5 children live in a county without a child psychiatrist, and only 35% of psychiatrists accept Medicaid.[52,53] Long distance appointments also mean that children are spending less time in school and caregivers are missing more time at work, both of which have significant consequences.

The increased number of children who are boarding in EDs and the increased length of time that they are staying have both psychological and economic costs. Youth have described the experience of boarding as traumatic and similar to incarceration.[17] Less than 20% of the youth who are boarding are receiving medication management or psychotherapy while they wait for psychiatric hospitalization.[17] Before 2020, median costs of youth mental health-related ED visits were steadily increasing.[54] The costs of staying less than 24 hours compared to more than 24 hours have a median difference of more than $3000.[54]

CHANGES IN TREATMENT APPROACHES

The increasing rate of psychiatric illness during the COVID-19 pandemic, seen particularly with depression and suicide, has forced the mental health landscape to make many changes to service delivery. Although there have been some initial concerns related to the impact of treatment effectiveness as a result of these changes, there are possible long-term benefits of these service delivery changes once key questions are answered.

The impact on care delivered in psychiatric inpatient units has been dramatic. For example, the pandemic requirement of the implementation of infection control measures led to a change in traditional milieu-based treatment approaches as well as a reduction of family and social visits.[43] Furthermore, there has been a loss of therapeutic groups and an alteration in the therapeutic milieu which has made the provision of care less optimal. Additionally, home-based care such as wraparound services, which historically mitigated the need for acute levels of care, was significantly impacted by the pandemic. Most of the services either ceased or were converted to telephone or video platforms, which diminished their benefits.[43]

Telehealth

One of the overarching treatment delivery adaptations to the COVID-19 pandemic has been the proliferation of treatment accessed via virtual platforms. There has been a growing body of literature focused on the treatment of pediatric anxiety supporting the delivery of cognitive behavioral therapy (CBT) using telehealth and virtual modalities.[55,56] Although less robust, there has also been evidence of the effectiveness of telehealth in targeting pediatric depression.[57] For example, data suggest that telehealth-based CBT used during the pandemic with youth with internalizing symptoms has been associated with significant reductions in youth depression.[58] Many advantages of the use of telehealth to deliver mental health treatment have been identified. Telehealth has been found to reduce unmet treatment needs especially in underserved areas. It also allows for treatment to occur amidst social distancing requirements, an important factor with the possibility of future viral outbreaks. The delivery of treatments in the home setting via telehealth also likely increases the ecological validity of those treatments, creating greater opportunity for maintenance and generalization of skills outside of the clinic.[57] CBT for the treatment of depression relies upon the assignment of behavioral strategies to practice between sessions; the ability to present and practice the skills in the target setting during telehealth sessions is increasingly useful.

Challenges to the use of telehealth in the treatment of pediatric depression have also been identified. First and foremost, although there has been a growing body of literature in support, research on the efficacy of assessment and treatment of pediatric depression via telehealth is still in its infancy. Much has been written about barriers to access. Low-income families, people of color, and rural communities still have less access to broadband Internet service and technological devices compared with more affluent non-Latinx White families.[59] Even when individuals have access to Internet connectivity, technological literacy may play a role in telehealth engagement. Such challenges may be especially important to consider for older individuals and families from linguistically diverse backgrounds accessing telehealth platforms that are not designed in their native language.[57] Additional challenges include reimbursement and legal barriers. As telehealth is becoming more commonplace, reimbursement for all mental health professionals is slowly coming online; however, variability across states still exists.[57] In addition, legal barriers include constraints related to state licensure and barriers related to the prescribing of certain medications.

Single Session Interventions

Given the extreme lack of mental health resources that has intensified during the pandemic, there has been a focus on freeing up treatment slots as quickly as possible. One such possibility is with single-session interventions. A recent randomized controlled trial (RCT) examining the efficacy of an online single-session intervention found symptom improvements in depression and hopelessness in a youth population.[60]

PROTECTIVE FACTORS AND AREAS FOR PREVENTION AND INTERVENTION

The US Surgeon General's report on youth mental health summarizes a multifaceted approach to supporting youth mental health.[61] The report emphasizes the importance of focusing on ensuring access to effective mental health care, creating environments in the school, home, and community that are supportive of positive mental health, and addressing societal factors that may contribute to poor mental health outcomes.[61]

Challenges with accessing mental health care, exacerbated during the COVID-19 pandemic, have increased the importance of identifying a range of approaches to delivering care.[62] Fortunately, there are opportunities for youth to obtain care in pediatric primary care and school settings, as well as more traditional behavioral health care settings. There are several advantages to making pediatric mental health care accessible through school and primary care settings, including obtaining care in settings that are familiar to children and families, integrating mental health with educational and health care teams, and the possibility of providing care before conditions have become more acute.

A common thread in prevention strategies for mental health issues is interpersonal connection. Relationships and a sense of belonging have a strong impact on both mental and physical health. Intentionally bolstering a "culture of connection" in places such as homes, clinics, schools, and communities is imperative for the health of people of all ages.[34]

Family Environment

The family environment is a key factor in contributing to positive mental health outcomes. Parents and caregivers play an important role in modeling effective strategies for coping with stress, as well as promoting healthy habits related to nutrition and sleep. Families can help youth establish and maintain routines such as attending school and extracurricular activities on a consistent basis, as well as facilitate opportunities for peer interactions to support development of healthy social relationships. Further, family members may serve as the initial people to recognize changes in their children that may require professional intervention.

A form of early prevention that families can implement is positive parenting techniques, which can improve emotional connectedness with parents and children and is associated with less depressive symptoms in adolescence.[63,64] There are multiple programs, such as Triple P, the Incredible Years, Everyday Parenting from Coursera, and Adults and Children Together Against Violence: Parents Raising Safe Kids Adults and Children Together (ACT), which teach similar evidence-based tenants of positive parenting. Core aspects include positive reinforcement, effective communication, selective ignoring, and logical consequences. Increasing dissemination and access to these techniques and programs could reduce future rates of depression.[65]

Family relationships and acceptance of children with an LGBTQ+ identity make a difference in mental health and substance-use health outcomes.[66] The more LGBTQ‾affirming environments that youth have, the less likely they are to make a suicide attempt.[67] Health care providers can provide evidence-based resources to families, such as from the Family Acceptance Project, that can help promote understanding and acceptance.[66]

Primary Care

Pediatric primary care is an important opportunity to increase access to mental health services, including identification and treatment of depression.[68] Families typically build relationships with primary health care teams over the course of their child's development, which may reduce barriers to early identification and intervention of psychiatric symptoms, as well as family acceptability of treatment recommendations.[69] Further, communication between mental health and medical clinicians can be more efficient in integrated care settings compared with more traditionally separated mental health and primary care settings. Systematic depression screening, particularly when integrated into an electronic health record, supports improvements in identification and rates of treatment of adolescent depression.[70] Pediatric health care systems should be encouraged and supported to continue expanding the integration of mental health screening, prevention, and intervention services in primary care settings.

To support pediatricians with the increasing demand for managing mental health conditions, there are expanding Pediatric Mental Health Care Access (PMHCA) Programs and collaborative care models (CoCMs), both of which have been shown to be effective strategies improving access to care.[71–74] PMHCA Programs, also known as Child Psychiatry Access Programs, typically provide access for pediatricians to

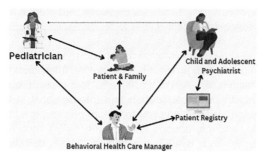

Fig. 6. CoCM multidisciplinary team. Solid arrows indicate close contact, dashed lines indicate infrequent communication. (*Source*: Figure was created using Canva.com.)

phone-based consultation with child and adolescent psychiatrists. The AAP has encouraged its local chapters to partner with PMHCA Programs, to facilitate pediatricians being able to provide care "sooner and with more confidence."[73] The CoCM involves a multidisciplinary team to support the patient, while receiving care from their pediatrician (**Fig. 6**). Once a pediatrician identifies a child or adolescent would benefit from mental health services, they are assigned a behavioral health care manager, who works closely with the patient and family to provide therapeutic interventions. The behavioral health care manager also reviews cases with a child and adolescent psychiatrist and communicates closely with the pediatrician. In the past few years, Centers for Medicare & Medicaid Services (CMS) has created billing codes for the CoCM, where the pediatrician bills for the services of the whole team. Currently, CoCM codes are covered by select state Medicaid programs and some private insurance plans.[74] The variable coverage has hindered expansion of CoCM programs; however, initial evidence is promising and as more payers provide reimbursement, the programs may become more available for pediatricians.

Schools

Schools also provide a familiar environment for adolescents in which mental health prevention and intervention efforts can be effectively integrated. Prior to the COVID-19 pandemic, approximately one-third of adolescents received mental health services through school-based programs.[75] Mental health support in a school setting starts with establishing an environment that is safe and affirming for a diverse range of students. A feeling of belonging and connection at school has been shown to be protective against development of mental health concerns.[76]

Schools are well positioned to recognize and respond to students who appear to struggle with coping with stress, demonstrating changes in their behavior or demeanor, or have unexpected absences or academic decline. The availability of mental health care in schools helps engage adolescents in treatment who may otherwise experience challenges obtaining effective services, as well as capitalize on the benefits of having access to input and support from teachers and other school professionals. School-based care decreases disparities in access relating to transportation and insurance.[77,78]

Schools are effective settings for the implementation of multi-tier models for universal support, screening, identification, and focused intervention.[79] School behavioral health services may be provided by a range of professionals, such as guidance counselors, school nurses, school social workers, and school psychologists.[80] School psychologists can have a particularly strong role with implementing depression interventions in school settings.[81] There is evidence that mental health support provided by school personnel has positive effects of academic, overall health, and mental health outcomes.[82]

In addition to being a venue for treatment, schools may provide an ideal setting for effective depression prevention programs, for example, Interpersonal Psychotherapy-Adolescent Skills Training (IPT-AST).[83,84] IPT-AST is a group-based prevention program that includes both psychoeducation and interpersonal skills building and is based on the theory that depression symptoms can be prevented by improving interpersonal relationships and interactions. Studies of IPT-AST support improvements in depression symptoms and overall functioning when compared with control groups.[83,84]

Historically, schools have had difficulty with obtaining adequate sustainable funding for specialized staff and mental health services. In May 2023, CMS released new comprehensive guidance for school-based Medicaid reimbursement for the first time in 20 years.[85] The update was designed to facilitate and encourage schools to utilize Medicaid as a funding source to sustainable reimburse for mental health services. States that have provided dedicated support for schools to optimize Medicaid reimbursement have seen increases in funding of tens of thousands of dollars, and up to doubling of their school behavioral health workforce.[86]

SUMMARY

The COVID-19 pandemic is a contributing factor to increasing rates of pediatric mental health, specifically depression and suicide. The far-reaching effects of the illness itself in addition to the public health response have both directly and indirectly led to increased symptoms of depression.[43]

The pre-existing shortcomings in the child and adolescent mental health system were overwhelmed during the pandemic, leading to insufficient access to care at every level, and escalating mental health emergencies, especially in minoritized groups. The pervasive effects of structural racism and socioeconomic disparities continue to cast a long shadow, and the resulting vulnerabilities were made acutely apparent during the COVID-19 pandemic. The ongoing disparities and upcoming Medicaid unwinding are part of the myriad of challenges adolescents still face in securing needed mental health services.

Our nation's youth are alarmingly in need, and there is a critical need for comprehensive, systemic, and sustainable interventions. Addressing these pressing concerns must be a top priority for pediatricians, child and adolescent psychiatrists, other mental health professionals, families, communities, and policymakers to safeguard the well-being and future of our current generation of children and adolescents.

CLINICS CARE POINTS

- In October 2021, the AAP, the AACAP and the CHA declared a national emergency in children's mental health, noting the multifold detrimental impact of the COVID-19 pandemic including adversity, disruption, loss of safety and structure, and disproportionate impacts on children of color due to structural racism.

- Social connection is intertwined with mental and physical health. Isolation and loneliness carry significant health risks and were exacerbated during the COVID-19 pandemic.

- The trends of increasing youth with mental health concerns worsened during the pandemic. In 2020, there was a 24% increase in ED visits for youth mental health concerns and in 2021, nearly a 51% increase in ED visits for suspected suicide attempts by teenage girls compared to 2019. This led to a boarding crisis, as there was a dearth of inpatient psychiatric hospital beds available for treatment of these youth, and medical hospitals were not equipped to treat youth with mental health crises.

- Certain minority youth were at higher risk during 2019 to 2021: Black and Hispanic youth had the steepest increases in feeling persistently sad and hopeless, and LGBTQ+ youth had the highest rates of suicidal ideation.

- Contributing factors to depression and suicidal ideation in adolescents include structural inequities, racial injustice, social isolation, adverse childhood experiences, and lack of or inadequate mental health care access.

- For support in providing mental health care to children and adolescents, pediatricians can engage with PMHCA Programs and CoCMs, which can improve confidence for pediatricians and increase access to mental health care services for young people.

- During the pandemic and after, there have been some innovations in health care delivery, which require more study and evidence. These include telehealth, single-session interventions, and consideration of evaluation and intervention in non-mental health settings, such as the family setting, the primary care setting, and the school setting.

DISCLOSURE

Drs J. Close and J. Lewis have no disclosures or conflicts to report. Dr S.H. Arshad has no conflicts, also receives funding from UC Irvine's Train New Trainer's program. Dr S.L. Soffer: Guilford Press (author). Dr T.D. Benton is on the AFSP Board, Friends Central School Board, and Juvenile Law Center Board, serves as AACAP President, and recieves NIH/PCORI funding.

FUNDING

Dr S.L. Soffer is the author of a book published by Guilford Press for which he receives royalties. Dr T.D. Benton is on the AFSP Board, Friends Central School Board, and Juvenile Law Center Board, serves as AACAP President, and recieves NIH/PCORI funding.

REFERENCES

1. American Academy of Pediatrics. American Academy of Child and Adolescent Psychiatry, Children's Hospital Association. AAP-AACAP-CHA Declaration of a National Emergency in Child and Adolescent Mental Health 2021. Available at: https://www.aap.org/en/advocacy/child-and-adolescent-healthy-mental-development/aap-aacap-cha-declaration-of-a-national-emergency-in-child-and-adolescent-mental-health/.
2. Hillis SD, Blenkinsop A, Villaveces A, et al. COVID-19–associated orphanhood and caregiver death in the United States. Pediatrics 2021;148(6).
3. Children's Hospital Association. Emergency room boarding of kids in mental health crisis. Available at: https://www.childrenshospitals.org/-/media/files/public-policy/mental_health/fact_sheets/boarding_fact_sheet_121421.pdf.
4. Whitney DG, Peterson MD. US National and State-Level Prevalence of Mental Health Disorders and Disparities of Mental Health Care Use in Children. JAMA Pediatr 2019;173(4):389–91.
5. Pradhan T, Six-Workman EA, Law KB. An innovative approach to care: integrating mental health services through telemedicine in rural school-based health centers. Psychiatr Serv 2019;70(3):239–42.

6. Kalb LG, Stapp EK, Ballard ED, et al. Trends in psychiatric emergency department visits among youth and young adults in the US. Pediatrics 2019;143(4).
7. Bommersbach TJ, McKean AJ, Olfson M, et al. National Trends in Mental Health-Related Emergency Department Visits Among Youth, 2011-2020. JAMA 2023; 329(17):1469–77.
8. CDC WONDER. Underlying Cause of Death, 1999-2020 Request. Available at: http://wonder.cdc.gov.
9. Joseph VA, Martínez-Alés G, Olfson M, et al. Temporal trends in suicide methods among adolescents in the US. JAMA Netw Open 2022;5(10):e2236049.
10. Farah R, Rege SV, Cole RJ, et al. Suspected suicide attempts by self-poisoning among persons aged 10–19 years during the COVID-19 pandemic — United States, 2020–2022. MMWR Morb Mortal Wkly Rep 2023;(72):426–30.
11. Mental Health America. The State of Mental Health in America 2023. 2023. Available at: https://mhanational.org/issues/2023/mental-health-america-youth-data.
12. Centers for Disease Control and Prevention. 10 leading causes of death, United States. Available at: https://wisqars.cdc.gov/data/lcd/home.
13. The White House. FACT SHEET: improving access and care for youth mental health and substance use conditions. 2021. Available at: https://www.whitehouse.gov/briefing-room/statements-releases/2021/10/19/fact-sheet-improving-access-and-care-for-youth-mental-health-and-substance-use-conditions/. [Accessed 23 August 2023].
14. Yard E, Radhakrishnan L, Ballesteros MF, et al. Emergency Department visits for suspected suicide attempts among persons aged 12–25 Years before and during the COVID-19 pandemic — United States, January 2019–may 2021. Centers for Disease Control and Prevention; 2021 (Morbidity and Mortality Weekly Report).
15. Centers for Disease Control and Prevention. Youth risk behavior survey data summary & trends report. 2021. Available at: https://www.cdc.gov/healthyyouth/data/yrbs/pdf/YRBS_Data-Summary-Trends_Report2023_508.pdf. [Accessed 17 October 2023].
16. Children's Hospital Association. The latest pediatric mental health data. 2023. Available at: https://www.childrenshospitals.org/news/childrens-hospitals-today/2023/04/the-latest-pediatric-mental-health-data.
17. Overhage L, Hailu R, Busch AB, et al. Trends in Acute Care Use for Mental Health Conditions Among Youth During the COVID-19 Pandemic. JAMA Psychiatr 2023; 80(9):924–32.
18. Horwitz SM, Storfer-Isser A, Kerker BD, et al. Barriers to the identification and management of psychosocial problems: changes from 2004 to 2013. Acad Pediatr 2015;15(6):613–20.
19. The Trevor Project. 2023 U.S. national survey on the mental health of LGBTQ young people. 2023. Available at: https://www.thetrevorproject.org/survey-2023/.
20. Kelly LM, Shepherd BF, Becker SJ. Elevated risk of substance use disorder and suicidal ideation among Black and Hispanic lesbian, gay, and bisexual adults. Drug Alcohol Depend 2021;226:108848.
21. Orris A, Wagner J. Medicaid School-Based Services Can Help Prevent "Unwinding" Coverage Losses. 2022. Available at: https://www.cbpp.org/blog/medicaid-school-based-services-can-help-prevent-unwinding-coverage-losses.
22. Álvarez B. Florida's New History Standard: 'A Blow to Our Students and Nation'. NEA Today 2023. Available at: https://www.nea.org/nea-today/all-news-articles/floridas-new-history-standard-blow-our-students-and-nation.
23. ACLU. Mapping Attacks on LGBTQ Rights in U.S. State Legislatures. Available at: https://www.aclu.org/legislative-attacks-on-lgbtq-rights.

24. Centers for Disease Control and Prevention. COVID Data Tracker. Available at: https://covid.cdc.gov/covid-data-tracker/#datatracker-home.
25. Romano S, Blackstock A, Taylor E, et al. Trends in Racial and Ethnic Disparities in COVID-19 Hospitalizations, by Region — United States, March–December 2020. MMWR Morb Mortal Wkly Rep 2021;(70):560–5.
26. Glower T. Uncovering COVID-19 disparities. Harvard Medical School News & Research; 2021. Available at: https://hms.harvard.edu/news/uncovering-covid-19-disparities.
27. Long KD, Albert SM. Use of zip code based aggregate indicators to assess race disparities in COVID-19. Ethn Dis. Summer 2021;31(3):399–406.
28. Trent M, Dooley DG, Dougé J, et al. The impact of racism on child and adolescent health. Pediatrics 2019;144(2).
29. Bor J, Venkataramani AS, Williams DR, et al. Police killings and their spillover effects on the mental health of black Americans: a population-based, quasi-experimental study. Lancet 2018;392(10144):302–10.
30. Lyn D. Timeline of Black Americans killed by police: 2014-2022. 2022. Available at: https://www.aa.com.tr/en/americas/timeline-of-black-americans-killed-by-police-2014-2022/2596913.
31. Centers for Disease Control and Prevention. New CDC data illuminate youth mental health threats during the COVID-19 pandemic. 2022. Available at: https://www.cdc.gov/media/releases/2022/p0331-youth-mental-health-covid-19.html.
32. Bryant M. 'It was time to take charge': the Black youth leading the George Floyd protests. 2020. Available at: https://www.theguardian.com/world/2020/jun/15/black-youth-activism-george-floyd-protests.
33. Almeida ILL, Rego JF, Teixeira ACG, et al. Social isolation and its impact on child and adolescent development: a systematic review. Rev Paul Pediatr 2021;40:e2020385.
34. Office of the Surgeon General. Our Epidemic of Loneliness and Isolation. The U.S. Surgeon General's Advisory on the Healing Effects of Social Connection and Community. 2023. Available at: https://www.hhs.gov/sites/default/files/surgeon-general-social-connection-advisory.pdf.
35. Bhogal A, Borg B, Jovanovic T, et al. Are the kids really alright? Impact of COVID-19 on mental health in a majority Black American sample of schoolchildren. Psychiatry Res 2021;304:114146.
36. Hoover S, Bostic J. Schools as a vital component of the child and adolescent mental health system. Psychiatr Serv 2021/01/01 2021;72(1):37–48.
37. Council on Criminal Justice. New Analysis Shows 8% Increase in U.S. Domestic Violence Incidents Following Pandemic Stay-At-Home Orders. Available at: https://counciloncj.org/new-analysis-shows-8-increase-in-u-s-domestic-violence-incidents-following-pandemic-stay-at-home-orders/.
38. American Academy of Child and Adolescent Psychiatry. Workforce Maps by state. Available at: https://www.aacap.org/aacap/Advocacy/Federal_and_State_Initiatives/Workforce_Maps/Home.aspx.
39. University of Michigan Behavioral Health Workforce Research Center. The child and adolescent psychologist workforce. 2020. Available at: https://www.behavioralhealthworkforce.org/wp-content/uploads/2020/07/Y5P3_The-Child-and-Adolescent-BH-Workforce_Full-Report.pdf.
40. America's school mental health report card. 2022. Available at: https://hopefulfutures.us/wp-content/uploads/2022/02/Final_Master_021522.pdf.

41. Goodman B. Long waiting lists, long drives and costly care hinder many kids' access to mental health care. 2022. Available at: https://www.cnn.com/2022/10/06/health/youth-parents-mental-health-kff-poll-wellness/index.html.
42. Pinals DA, Hepburn B, Parks J, et al. The behavioral health system and its response to COVID-19: a snapshot perspective. Psychiatr Serv 2020;71(10):1070–4.
43. Cama SF, Miyamoto BE, DeJong SM. Impact on child psychiatry. Psychiatr Clin North Am 2022;45(1):133–46.
44. The Joint Commission. Patient flow through the emergency department. 2012. *R3 Report*. Available at: https://www.jointcommission.org/standards/r3-report/r3-report-issue-4-patient-flow-through-the-emergency-department/.
45. McEnany FB, Ojugbele O, Doherty JR, et al. Pediatric mental health boarding. Pediatrics 2020;146(4).
46. Cutler GJ, Bergmann KR, Doupnik SK, et al. Pediatric Mental Health Emergency Department Visits and Access to Inpatient Care: A Crisis Worsened by the COVID-19 Pandemic. Acad Pediatr 2022;22(6):889–91.
47. Leeb RT, Bitsko RH, Radhakrishnan L, et al. Mental Health-Related Emergency Department Visits Among Children Aged <18 Years During the COVID-19 Pandemic - United States, January 1-October 17, 2020. MMWR Morb Mortal Wkly Rep 2020;69(45):1675–80.
48. Perrin JM, Asarnow JR, Stancin T, et al. Mental Health Conditions and Health Care Payments for Children with Chronic Medical Conditions. Acad Pediatr 2019;19(1):44–50.
49. Doupnik SK, Rodean J, Feinstein J, et al. Health Care Utilization and Spending for Children With Mental Health Conditions in Medicaid. Acad Pediatr 2020;20(5):678–86.
50. 20,000% Increase for Employers: Youth Mental Health Telehealth Costs Soar Amid Double-Digit Jumps in Diagnoses, Suicide Attempts. Businesswire a Berkshire Hathaway Company. Available at: https://www.businesswire.com/news/home/20221208005181/en/20000-Increase-for-Employers-Youth-Mental-Health-Teleheal th-Costs-Soar-Amid-Double-Digit-Jumps-in-Diagnoses-Suicide-Attempts.
51. The White House. Reducing the economic burden of unmet mental health needs. 2022. Available at: https://www.whitehouse.gov/cea/written-materials/2022/05/31/reducing-the-economic-burden-of-unmet-mental-health-needs/.
52. McBain RK, Kofner A, Stein BD, et al. Growth and distribution of child psychiatrists in the United States: 2007-2016. Pediatrics 2019;144(6).
53. Wen H, Wilk AS, Druss BG, et al. Medicaid acceptance by psychiatrists before and after medicaid expansion. JAMA Psychiatr 2019;76(9):981–3.
54. Hoffmann JA, Stack AM, Samnaliev M, et al. Trends in Visits and Costs for Mental Health Emergencies in a Pediatric Emergency Department, 2010-2016. Acad Pediatr May-Jun 2019;19(4):386–93.
55. Hill C, Creswell C, Vigerland S, et al. Navigating the development and dissemination of internet cognitive behavioral therapy (iCBT) for anxiety disorders in children and young people: A consensus statement with recommendations from the #iCBTLorentz Workshop Group. Internet Interv 2018;12:1–10.
56. Shirotsuki K, Sugaya N, Nakao M. Descriptive review of internet-based cognitive behavior therapy on anxiety-related problems in children under the circumstances of COVID-19. Biopsychosoc Med 2022;16(1):3.
57. Ros-DeMarize R, Chung P, Stewart R. Pediatric behavioral telehealth in the age of COVID-19: Brief evidence review and practice considerations. Curr Probl Pediatr Adolesc Health Care 2021;51(1):100949.

58. Uysal B, Morgül E, Taştekne F, et al. Videoconferencing-based cognitive behavioral therapy for youth with anxiety and depression during COVID-19 pandemic. Sch Psychol Int 2022;43(4):420–39.
59. Chavira DA, Ponting C, Ramos G. The impact of COVID-19 on child and adolescent mental health and treatment considerations. Behav Res Ther 2022;157: 104169.
60. Schleider JL, Mullarkey MC, Fox KR, et al. A randomized trial of online single-session interventions for adolescent depression during COVID-19. Nat Hum Behav 2022;6(2):258–68.
61. Office of the Surgeon General. Protecting youth mental health: the U.S. Surgeon General's Advisory. 2021. Available at: https://www.hhs.gov/sites/default/files/surgeon-general-youth-mental-health-advisory.pdf.
62. Lewandowski RE, O'Connor B, Bertagnolli A, et al. Screening for and diagnosis of depression among adolescents in a large health maintenance organization. Psychiatr Serv 2016;67(6):636–41.
63. Keijser R, Olofsdotter S, Nilsson KW, et al. The influence of parenting styles and parental depression on adolescent depressive symptoms: A cross-sectional and longitudinal approach. Mental Health & Prevention 2020;20:200193.
64. Webster-Stratton C, Herman KC. The impact of parent behavior-management training on child depressive symptoms. J Counsel Psychol 2008;55(4):473–84.
65. Fortson BL, Klevens J, Merrick MT, et al. Preventing child abuse and neglect: a technical package for policy, norm, and programmatic activities. 2016. Available at: https://www.cdc.gov/violenceprevention/pdf/can-prevention-technical-package.pdf.
66. Ryan C, Huebner D, Diaz RM, et al. Family rejection as a predictor of negative health outcomes in white and latino lesbian, gay, and bisexual young adults. Pediatrics 2009;123(1):346–52.
67. The Trevor Project. The Trevor Project research Brief: LGBTQ & gender-affirming Spaces. 2020. Available at: https://www.thetrevorproject.org/wp-content/uploads/2021/07/LGBTQ-Affirming-Spaces_-December-2020.pdf.
68. Asarnow JR, Miranda J. Improving care for depression and suicide risk in adolescents: innovative strategies for bringing treatments to community settings. Annu Rev Clin Psychol 2014;10:275–303.
69. Cheung AH, Kozloff N, Sacks D. Pediatric depression: an evidence-based update on treatment interventions. Curr Psychiatr Rep 2013;15(8):381.
70. Farley AM, Gallop RJ, Brooks ES, et al. Identification and management of adolescent depression in a large pediatric care network. J Dev Behav Pediatr Feb/2020; 41(2):85–94.
71. Clinical Update: collaborative mental health care for children and adolescents in pediatric primary care. J Am Acad Child Adolesc Psychiatry 2023;62(2):91–119.
72. Sullivan K, George P, Horowitz K. Addressing National Workforce Shortages by Funding Child Psychiatry Access Programs. Pediatrics 2021;147(1).
73. American Academy of Pediatrics. Tips for AAP Chapters: Increasing Access to Behavioral Health Care via Telehealth by Partnering with Pediatric Mental Health Care Access Programs. 2021. Available at: https://www.aap.org/en/practice-management/care-delivery-approaches/telehealth/increasing-access-to-behavioral-health-care-via-telehealth-by-partnering-with-pediatric-mental-health-care-access-programs/.
74. Meadows Mental Health Policy Institute, The Commonwealth Fund. Improving behavioral health care for youth through collaborative care expansion. 2022. Available at: https://mmhpi.org/wp-content/uploads/2022/11/Behavioral-Health-Care-for-Youth-CoCM-Expansion-Nov2022.pdf.

75. Ali MM, West K, Teich JL, et al. Utilization of mental health services in educational setting by adolescents in the United States. J Sch Health 2019;89(5):393–401.
76. Breedlove M, Choi J, Zyromski B. Mitigating the effects of adverse childhood experiences: how restorative practices in schools support positive childhood experiences and protective factors. N Educat 2021;17(3):223–41.
77. Hoffmann JA, Alegría M, Alvarez K, et al. Disparities in pediatric mental and behavioral health conditions. Pediatrics 2022;(4):150.
78. So M, McCord RF, Kaminski JW. Policy levers to promote access to and utilization of children's mental health services: a systematic review. Adm Pol Ment Health 2019;46(3):334–51.
79. National Association of School Psychologists. Appropriate Behavioral, Social, and Emotional Supports to Meet the Needs of All Students (Position Statement). 2009.
80. Mellin EA, Anderson-Butcher D, Bronstein LR. Strengthening interprofessional team collaboration: potential roles for school mental health professionals. Advances in School Mental Health Promotion 2011;4:51–60.
81. Splett JW, Fowler J, Weist MD, et al. The critical role of school psychology in the school mental health movement. Psychol Sch 2013;50(3):245–58.
82. Close J, Schmal S, Essick E, et al. Specialized Instructional Support Personnel (SISP): A Promising Solution for North Carolina's Youth Mental Health Crisis. N C Med J 2023;84(5).
83. Young JF, Benas JS, Schueler CM, et al. A Randomized Depression Prevention Trial Comparing Interpersonal Psychotherapy–Adolescent Skills Training to Group Counseling in Schools. Prev Sci 2016;17(3):314–24.
84. Young JF, Mufson L, Davies M. Efficacy of Interpersonal Psychotherapy-Adolescent Skills Training: an indicated preventive intervention for depression. J Child Psychol Psychiatry 2006;47(12):1254–62.
85. Centers for Medicare & Medicaid Services. Delivering Services in School-Based Settings: A Comprehensive Guide to Medicaid Services and Administrative Claiming 2023. Available at: https://www.medicaid.gov/medicaid/financial-management/downloads/sbs-guide-medicaid-services-administrative-claiming.pdf. [Accessed 23 August 2023].
86. Healthy Schools Campaign. Financial Impact of Expanding School Medicaid Programs. 2022. Available at: https://healthystudentspromisingfutures.org/wp-content/uploads/2022/07/Financial-Impact-of-Expanding-School-Medicaid.pdf. [Accessed 17 October 2023].

The Impact of COVID on Adolescent Anxiety

Trends, Clinical Considerations, and Treatment Recommendations

Izabela Milaniak, PhD*, Stephanie Davidson, MD,
Bruce Leewiwatanakul, DO, Tami D. Benton, MD

KEYWORDS

• Anxiety • Adolescents • COVID • Anxiety disorders • Social anxiety • OCD • GAD

KEY POINTS

- Rates of clinical anxiety symptoms in youth have increased during COVID and post-quarantine.
- Increased rates are likely due to adaptive threat calibration and reinforcement of avoidance patterns due to quarantine.
- Hybrid utilization of in-person and telehealth services is uniquely suited for the treatment of anxiety disorders.
- Given the gap in behavioral health medical and behavioral treatment providers, it is recommended that alternative treatment settings such as school and primary care be utilized.

INTRODUCTION

In December 2019, coronavirus (COVID) emerged and rapidly spread globally. By Spring 2020, most of the world had implemented quarantine measures, keeping youth and caregivers home from school and work. For upwards of 2 years, children and adolescents were removed from their typical environments and life shifted to a primarily virtual existence. In addition, COVID acted as an accelerant to societal, economic, and political tensions that had already reached a zenith prior to the pandemic. Media coverage of deaths, overtaxed health systems, and traumatized health care workers was interspersed with footage of police brutality subsequent Black Lives Matter protests often resulting in violence against protestors. COVID fanned flames of political

Perelman School of Medicine at the University of Pennsylvania, Children's Hospital of Philadelphia, CHOP Center for Advanced Behavioral Healthcare, 4601 Market Street, Third Floor, Philadelphia, PA 19139, USA
* Corresponding author. CHOP Center for Advanced Behavioral Healthcare, 4601 Market Street, Third Floor, Philadelphia, PA 19139.
E-mail address: milaniaki@chop.edu

Pediatr Clin N Am 71 (2024) 601–612
https://doi.org/10.1016/j.pcl.2024.04.003
0031-3955/24/© 2024 Elsevier Inc. All rights reserved.
pediatric.theclinics.com

ideologies based in xenophobia, racism, misogyny, homophobia, and transphobia, and increased violence against these minoritized populations, in the context of unprecedented levels of economic inequality worldwide. Pre-pandemic, youth mental health was already reaching crisis level, and exposure to these serious threats to young people's sense of safety and well-being, understandably exacerbated this crisis. Now in 2024, although COVID is far from a distant concern, society has mostly returned to routine life. However, the youth mental health crisis has not subsided. Children and adolescents are given the incredibly difficult task of not only recovering from the past few years and re-entering every-day life, but also of finding a way forward in an increasingly uncertain world, as they try to build a future for themselves. In this article, the authors discuss the role COVID had on recalibrating youth's experience of threat to begin understanding how mechanisms of fear and anxiety in youth in a post-quarantine world can pave a path for resilience and recovery.

Anxiety and related disorders (ARDs) are the most common mental health diagnoses in youth and include social anxiety disorder, separation anxiety disorder, generalized anxiety disorder (GAD), obsessive compulsive disorder (OCD) and so on. Predictably, rates of clinically elevated symptoms of anxiety increased during the pandemic. One meta-analysis of over 80,000 youth globally, reported that the prevalence of clinical generalized anxiety symptoms in the population, including uncontrollable worry and hyperarousal, nearly doubled (from 11.6% to 20.5%) compared with pre-pandemic estimates and that prevalence rates continued to increase as the pandemic continued.[1] A meta-analysis of longitudinal studies assessing changes in anxiety levels within individuals reported an increase in clinical anxiety symptoms, even when controlling for pre-pandemic baseline anxiety.[2] Understandably, the pandemic environment exacerbated anxiety in youth who were already struggling; however, COVID also pushed many youth who were at-risk but maintaining function and even youth with minimal or no anxiety disorder histories or risk factors, into developing clinically significant levels of anxiety. Longitudinal research on youth anxiety trajectories during COVID showed the steepest increase in clinical anxiety in adolescents with the lowest pre-pandemic levels of anxiety or those who were recovering/in remission from anxiety disorders prior to the pandemic.[3]

Similar to pre-pandemic estimates, meta-analytic data showed that adolescent girls continue to be the most vulnerable group for anxiety during and post-quarantine. In addition, rates of increased clinical anxiety were much higher in samples with higher proportions of racial and ethnic minoritized groups (40% in minoritized compared to 12%). LGBTQI youth were also particularly vulnerable to effects of COVID, as quarantine increased their proximity to unsupportive family members during an alarming increase in anti-LGBTQI legislation and social discourse. For example, LGBTQI college students experienced a doubling of severe psychological distress from pre-pandemic levels (26%–43%) with significant increases in sexual and gender identity-related distress, and higher levels of hiding their identities due to experiencing more negative comments.[4] Overall, data suggest that youth with the following characteristics remain the most vulnerable for clinical anxiety and should be especially considered for identification and intervention: (1) older adolescent, (2) female gender, (3) minoritized racial identity, and (4) queer sexual and/or gender identity.

BACKGROUND

Understanding the profound effect that COVID had on youth anxiety first requires an understanding of how the anxiety system functions normatively. Fear by itself is an efficient survival strategy, as the brain automatically processes and responds to environmental threats without needing slow, conscious processing that would delay the rapid fight–flight–freeze response and lower the chance of survival. Humans have the additional advantage of anxiety, the anticipation of future threats, allowing us to prepare for imagined threats ahead of time—a process we describe as worry. Fear and anxiety/worry are normal, natural, adaptive, and essential processes that not only keep us safe but also help motivate us into action as members of a communal society. Fear/anxiety is our brain's threat identification, processing, and response system that dynamically recalibrates in response to experiential learning. ARDs happen when our brain's threat system becomes miscalibrated and stuck in a rigid, negatively biased processing style, causing overestimation of the likelihood and intensity of threats and underestimation of one's threat-management capabilities.

This negatively biased threat calibration is strengthened and reinforced through continuous learning from behavioral responses to threats—typically increasing compulsive avoidance of situations that trigger the ever-expanding repertoire of potential threats. The more people avoid safe situations their threat system erroneously coded as dangerous, the more that miscalibration solidifies and, with continued avoidance, anxiety grows as perceived threats grow. Avoidance is the main behavioral mechanism and inflexibility the main cognitive mechanism by which normative levels of anxiety can transform into a disorder. Therefore, avoidance and inflexibility are the main treatment targets in evidence-based ARD treatments like cognitive behavioral therapy (CBT) and acceptance and commitment therapy (ACT). Because the threat system is primarily recalibrated through experience, behavioral intervention in the form of exposures to feared situations and prevention of avoidant responses is the "essential ingredient" in ARD treatments.

TRENDS IN CLINICAL ANXIETY
Threat Calibration

Given these two central mechanisms (experiential avoidance and inflexible overextension of threat) involved in ARDs, it is easy to see why a global mass casualty event like COVID, and its societal ramifications, has had such profound effects on youth's development of clinical anxiety. This is especially relevant to adolescent populations, as adolescence represents a second sensitive period of brain development during which calibration of the threat system is particularly salient and has the potential to be more entrenched. As the age group that was the most online during the pandemic, the adolescent brain was bombarded with an unprecedented volume of threatening imagery and content in the digital age of 24/7 news and social media cycles where exposure was inescapable and relentless. Mass confusion and rampant misinformation clouded the true nature of threats, leading to increased uncertainty about how to respond. A recent review of several studies showed increases in clinical anxiety in youth were higher in those with greater consumption of COVID-related news, especially in youth reporting high levels of uncertainty about validity of information.[5] It is therefore important for adolescents, especially those prone to anxiety, to limit exposure to negative news, including setting aside specific times for news updates to avoid excessive "doomscrolling." Furthermore, it is imperative to educate youth on critical media consumption, including spotting misinformation and recognizing fear mongering or sensationalized presentation of events.

While rising rates of clinical anxiety during and post-quarantine are concerning, it is important to not over-pathologize adaptive threat responses. Arguably, an increase in anxiety during a genuinely threatening and uncertain time was and continues to be a functional adaptation to an increasingly threatening and unpredictable environment. Increased threat hypervigilance undoubtedly influenced youth to appropriately socially distance, wear masks, and follow Centers for Disease Control and Prevention guidelines to keep safe. One could argue being *not anxious enough* during quarantine put youth and others at greater risk. Additionally, continuing high rates of anxiety post-quarantine can also be perceived as adaptive considering that the threat of COVID and the societal, economic, and political ramifications are still ongoing.

In the path forward, it is extremely important to conceptualize and treat anxiety in youth from a more balanced perspective, evaluating the adaptiveness and functionality of symptoms, rather than automatically labeling them as exaggerated. In today's world, previously unlikely situations (eg, pandemics, school shootings, terrorist attacks, war, climate change/severe weather patterns, political upheaval) are not perceived as low likelihood events, especially when reminders of these threats are inescapable. This is relevant particularly to worries and behaviors regarding safety, illness, contamination, and the future in which increased anxiety as a result of global shared experiences (eg, quarantine) but also individual histories (eg, having a family member pass away due to COVID) is functional and can lead to greater awareness of threats and subsequent reasonable preparation to adequately face them. On the other hand, anxiety becomes nonfunctional when preparatory behavior for threats is disproportionate to its likelihood (eg, not going to school at all for fear of school shootings), excessive (eg, washing hands for 15 minutes after potential contamination), or ineffective/inefficient (eg, ruminating without coping). In today's world, helping adolescents assess the usefulness of worrying patterns, rather than their rationality, may be a more effective strategy. Cognitive strategies targeting the irrationality of anxious thoughts, such as cognitive restructuring, should be reserved for clearly nonfunctional applications of anxiety. When applied to increased anxiety that makes sense given a threatening environment, this can be perceived as dismissive and invalidating, especially in vulnerable populations often encountering unsafe situations. In addition to "traditional" CBT techniques such as cognitive restructuring and exposures, clinicians should utilize third-wave CBT techniques (eg, ACT, DBT, and mindfulness), focusing on acceptance of uncertainty and lack of control, importance of values, and development of distress tolerance and thought distancing to help cope with their real experiences rather than try to convince them their fears are irrational.

Experiential Avoidance

Compared to diagnoses like GAD, illness anxiety, and contamination OCD, in which the line between functional and nonfunctional calibration of threat is blurred in the post-quarantine environment, social anxiety more clearly demonstrates COVID increasing levels of nonfunctional anxiety. The pandemic environment with quarantine, work and school closures, online schooling, social distancing, and avoidance of nonessential social interactions represents a very profound and prolonged example of (involuntary) avoidance of daily social life and interaction. Given that adolescence is an integral stage of social and emotional development, during which peers are the most significant source of social development and support, COVID posed a major interruption to youth social and emotional development. As previously mentioned, chronic avoidance of an environmental trigger (eg, social interactions), recalibrates the threat system to interpret the trigger as inherently threatening, escalating anxious physiologic and cognitive responses to that situation. With increased social avoidance, the brain generalizes threat to more types of social experiences as dangerous and shrinks the adolescent's social world. The brain also "learns" through repeated avoidant responding, that the adolescent is incapable of managing social situations effectively, decreasing sense of social efficacy, compounded by deteriorating (or underdevelopment of) social skills in the face of avoidance.

As social anxiety disorder typically develops around age 13 to 14 years, social isolation due to COVID likely significantly impacted social anxiety via mechanisms of avoidance by (1) exacerbating existing pre-pandemic social anxiety symptoms in the post-quarantine period; (2) converting mild social anxiety symptoms pre-pandemic to a full-blown disorder; and (3) developing new social anxiety symptoms in adolescents without histories of social anxiety. Because avoidance often results in short-term relief but long-term increases in anxiety, it is likely that for youth with pre-existing social anxiety, initial quarantine orders resulted in relief and temporary functional improvements.[6] However, following prolonged avoidance, the return to school, work, extracurriculars, and general daily social life was jarring for many adolescents. Anecdotal clinical experience describes increased difficulty in adjusting to post-quarantine social expectations and higher rates of school resistance and refusal, even in adolescents who did not previously struggle with social anxiety or school refusal. Research shows not all youth returned to consistent in-person schooling post-quarantine and chronic school absenteeism is at an all-time high.[7] Rates of chronic school absenteeism (eg, missing more than 10% of the school year) doubled from 8 million pre-pandemic to 16 million in 2022, disproportionately affecting Latino, black, and low-income youth. Concerningly, chronically absent students are more likely to fall behind and/or drop out.

Chronic absenteeism is likely the culmination of many factors stemming from the pandemic. Increased levels of anxiety related to social settings, contamination, and illness concerns likely impact absenteeism, as the brain has recalibrated school/socialization as inherently dangerous and necessary to avoid. For adolescents continuing to struggle with re-integration into their social environments and school/social avoidance, an exposure framework is necessary to encourage approach behaviors to recalibrate the school environment as safe. Although necessary early in the pandemic, virtual/online schooling feeds into the avoidance cycle and anxious adolescents should be encouraged to attend in-person schooling as much as possible, barring specific safety concerns or cultural/familial values around home-schooling. For those homeschooling for other reasons, it is imperative that social needs that would otherwise be met in school, are explicitly addressed. Developmentally, school serves as the primary setting for normative social and emotional development, and given this major interruption, it is likely that resulting social skill deficits and perceptions of social self-efficacy play a larger role in social anxiety presentations than ever before. Subsequently, special attention should be paid to actual versus perceived social skill deficits in adolescents with social anxiety, with intervention emphasizing building social self-efficacy to meet social challenges. As with threats regarding safety and illness, it is important to assess whether adolescents have a history of bullying by peers or community violence that resulted in past or current functional social avoidance for safety. If so, a trauma-informed approach that might include processing past events first or safety planning if threats are ongoing, may be necessary to improve socialization while maintaining safety.

TREATMENT CONSIDERATIONS AND RECOMMENDATIONS

Even prior to the pandemic, there has been a growing gap between the prevalence of common mental health conditions in youth and the availability of and access to appropriate evidence-based treatments, including a continued pediatric behavioral health (BH) specialist shortage. As the COVID pandemic both worsened anxiety symptoms for symptomatic youth and increased symptoms for youth in remission or without anxiety disorders, disproportion between demand for services and a health care infrastructure to meet these needs has increased greatly. It is therefore imperative that caregivers and health care providers think creatively about how evidence-based treatments can be delivered in alternate ways and alternate settings. We discuss several options for innovative treatment delivery options including telehealth, primary care (PC), and school-based care.

Telehealth

Shifting BH treatment to telehealth during COVID out of necessity represents one of the biggest shifts in therapeutic practice in recent history. Prior to the pandemic, almost all treatment options for ARDs were provided in-person and although available, telehealth therapy was not routinely practiced as it is now. It is important to realize how rapidly the adoption of telehealth needed to happen in response to COVID. As a result, health systems, training programs, clinicians, and researchers did not have a comprehensive, pre-existing understanding of best practices for telehealth-based mental health treatment. For ARDs in youth, meta-analysis of randomized control trial data shows telehealth and in-person versions of evidence-based treatments for ARDs in youth are equally effective.[8] However, more data are needed to make better person-centered clinical care decisions regarding telehealth for anxiety, such as who gets telehealth for which types of anxiety presentations, when, and how.

In addition, standard practice for ARD treatment appears to have settled on a hybrid model (eg, some in-person and some telehealth sessions). However, studies have only compared exclusively in-person or virtual treatments. To our knowledge, there is no empirical research examining hybrid model effectiveness, even though its flexibility may provide the best patient-centered care. For ARDs, in particular, telehealth not only can be *as good* as in-person care but may be *better* in certain presentations with certain patient/family characteristics. A fantastic review of clinical guidelines for telehealth for ARDs, Islam and colleagues[9] discussed advantages and disadvantages for telehealth and clinical guidelines around visit-type decisions. Researchers discussed increased access and ecological validity of the exposure environment (eg, exposure to "contaminated" home spaces) as the main advantage of telehealth-based exposures, but less oversight of the environment as the main disadvantage.

The promise of telehealth has historically focused on increasing access and removing barriers of in-person care including transportation, childcare, location/distance, and busy schedules, assuming services could reach minoritized populations historically unable to access care.[10] However, although racially minoritized youth were at greater risk for clinically significant levels of anxiety, data from several large pediatric health systems unfortunately demonstrated that transition to telehealth actually increased racial disparities in BH care access, particularly in urban areas.[11] The proportion of non-white pediatric patients decreased, and white patients increased. Digital disparities (eg, internet/smartphone access, digital literacy) likely influenced this trend; however, it is important to not conclude that this was the sole factor. Health systems should not underestimate the power of in-person interaction to build trust between a largely white provider base and minoritized populations that understandably are distrustful of a system that has historically caused harm to their communities. Research shows that black caregivers expressed more concerns about telehealth than White caregivers based on privacy, confidentiality, and physical absence of the provider.[12] Given that pre-COVID, non-white populations were already less likely to access mental health services due to stigma and mistrust, it is important to consider the potential effects of telehealth on the therapeutic alliance. Exposure-based ARD treatment heavily relies on the trust and buy-in of caregivers/youth as the provider must therapeutically temporarily increase anxiety and other challenging emotions during the session. Providers must pay special attention to family/patient factors that may make treatment *less* accessible through telehealth, including digital disparities and language proficiency. Providers must assess patient and family comfort level, ensuring home environments have safe spaces where adolescents can speak freely without privacy or confidentiality concerns. In-person sessions early in treatment should be considered to build therapeutic alliance, trust, and comfort and/or intermittent in-person sessions to maintain the relationship. Youth should be asked how comfortable or safe they feel in treatment at home and routinely confirm whether they are alone and/or able to speak freely during sessions.

Focus on access to care should be followed by assessing the quality and effectiveness of the accessed services, especially since treatment drop-out rates are high in youth, and higher in minoritized populations.[13] Because empirical data on telehealth effectiveness for different populations and clinical presentations are sparse, it is unclear whether telehealth dilutes important factors such as therapeutic alliance and treatment engagement that have historically be shown to be integral in treatment effectiveness. Research shows that the odds of appointment nonattendance for youth behavioral telehealth visits were nearly 4 times greater than for in-person visits.[14] Telehealth fundamentally changes the treatment setting and may result in sessions feeling more optional than in-person services. This is particularly relevant for adolescents, as parents may be less involved and not even present for telehealth sessions since they do not need to provide transportation. Given that telehealth alone impacts treatment attendance, youth with ARD who are prone to avoidance strategies are at a higher risk to disengage from treatment when nonattendance is easier. This is crucial during the exposure phase of treatment, as increased exposure practice leads to faster and more successful progress and missed sessions can undermine the momentum of approach behaviors and reignite avoidance strategies, especially in patients who struggle practicing exposures independently outside of sessions.

Considerations regarding whether telehealth may inadvertently reinforce avoidance in anxious youth, begs the question of which ARD presentations and comorbidities are more conducive to telehealth versus in-person visits. One must weigh the benefits of ecological validity of exposures done in the home environment with the costs of reduced provider and caregivers control over avoidance/exposure refusal or safety behaviors during exposures. Therefore, the extent to which targets are triggered more effectively in non-office environments versus the extent of avoidance, readiness, and willingness to break avoidance should guide the decision around visit types. Based on this, anxiety diagnoses that do not routinely require exposures such as GAD and anxiety presentations requiring more cognitive and/or emotional work, are likely to be more successful in telehealth. Telehealth has the potential to innovate and improve treatment outcomes for contamination and just right presentations of OCD, as the adolescent's bedroom, bathroom, and personal items are often the most powerful exposure targets and are only accessible via telehealth visits. In office exposures often suffer from lack of generalization to other environments, which reduce their power to recalibrate the threat-response system more comprehensively.

However, for targets involving social situations (eg, social anxiety, panic disorder, vomit phobia, OCD fears of contamination from others), in-person sessions can act as powerful naturalistic exposures, as patients must navigate several perceived threats to attend (eg, other people, transportation, crowds), and virtual sessions may allow for increased avoidance through the screen, being off-camera, or turning off the camera. As a result, it is generally recommended that social anxiety treatments have as much in-person treatment as possible—especially given the prolonged period of COVID-related social avoidance. Telehealth can be effective for socially related exposures, for example, if the patient is prompted to enter social situations, but the provider has less control in maintaining patient safety and privacy and requires additional informed consent from youth and their caregivers. Finally, comorbid conditions, most notably attention deficit hyperactivity disorder (ADHD) may make telehealth treatment for anxiety particularly challenging and make more frequent in-person sessions necessary. Executive dysfunction including difficulty paying attention and distractibility are more prevalent at home, and directly impact absorption of treatment interventions. The tool in which treatment is delivered (laptop, phone) by itself is a tempting distraction during the session, especially for teens who spend the most time on their phones and on social media.

In conclusion, the ideal candidates for telehealth ARD treatment are adolescents with good executive functioning skills, minimal levels of resistance, mild-to-moderate levels of avoidance, requiring less exposure-heavy treatment or external-world exposures and with acceptable levels of treatment engagement, especially motivation for exposures. Decision-making regarding treatment modality for ARDs must balance costs and benefits, including easier access versus lower engagement and more naturalistic environment versus less control. Decisions should be made collaboratively by providers, patients, and their families based on the likelihood of successful intervention and visit type should be dynamically assessed throughout treatment and adjusted as necessary.

School-based Services

While telehealth can expand the reach of pediatric BH providers, there is still an underlying national shortages of mental health specialists for youth. It is therefore vital that caregivers and clinicians be aware of innovations in alternative settings for delivery of mental health treatment outside of traditional specialist outpatient settings that are currently managing high volumes of referrals without a sufficient workforce to address the surge, leading to long waitlists and treatment delays. In fact, research shows that schools in the United States are now more common mental health care sites for youth (22%), when compared to traditional outpatient settings (20%).[15] A recent meta-analysis examining 29 RCTs for school-based interventions showed a positive effect, especially for the treatment of anxiety and CBT-based approaches to intervention.[16] This makes sense given that school environments are often the most common triggers for ARDs (eg, test and academic anxiety, social anxiety, contamination fears) and in-school interventions can have high levels of ecological validity. Interestingly, only clinician-delivered school-based programs had positive effects; teacher-delivered programs were ineffective. In addition, interventions at school were more effective for middle and high school populations compared to elementary school, suggesting that school-based intervention for ARD may be particularly efficacious for adolescents. Importantly, there was no difference between short-term versus long-term interventions suggesting that even brief interventions in schools can be effective and that longer term treatment may not be necessary for everyone. In addition to inquiring about formal school-based interventions for anxiety, patients, caregivers, and providers are encouraged to work with school staff to help manage student anxiety during the school day, especially if anxiety is interfering with academic, social, and emotional functioning while at school. Section 504 plans for anxiety disorders are highly recommended and should create a balance between accommodation of anxiety (eg, being able to take breaks) without reinforcing avoidance (eg, must return to class after break). Working with school staff is especially important for youth with school resistance or refusal due to anxiety, where gradual re-entry to the school environment is necessary.

Primary Care

PC has been called the "de facto" BH system in the United States, especially in pediatric populations where around half of PC visits are due to a BH or educational concern[17] and 85% of psychotropic medication for youth is managed by a primary care provider (PCP). This is especially relevant as COVID exacerbated the ongoing national shortage of child and adolescent psychiatrists (CAPs), with an estimated 14 CAPs per 100,000 children.[18] The American Academy of Pediatrics stance is that PCPs should have a major role in screening, assessment, and pharmacologic treatment of youth mental health concerns and developed a toolkit to assist PCPs.[19] The US Preventive Services Task Force has recommended that youth over the age of 7 years be routinely screened for anxiety in the PC setting.[20] Given the CAP service gap, it is recommended that PCPs initiate and manage medication in mild-to-moderate anxiety presentations and/or single diagnosis cases, and reserve referrals to CAPs for severe anxiety, complex comorbid BH concerns (eg, autism, ADHD), and/or complex chronic health conditions where considerations of drug interactions may necessitate more specialty care.

To aid in decision making for ARD in youth, PCPs are directed to the American Academy of Child and Adolescent Psychiatrists (AACAP) clinical practice guidelines for screening, assessment, and pharmacologic treatment.[21] The first-line medication recommended is selective serotonin reuptake inhibitors (SSRIs), typically sertraline, fluoxetine, and escitalopram. The main mechanism of action for all SSRIs is binding to the serotonin transporter and inhibiting reuptake of serotonin which leaves more of it in the synaptic cleft, while they are differentiated by their secondary actions on receptors for other neurotransmitters (eg, norepinephrine). Extensive research has shown that a combination of SSRI treatment and CBT to be more effective than either alone (though both CBT and SSRIs are effective on their own) and therefore the AACAP recommends combination treatment for moderate-to-severe anxiety presentations, while therapy alone for mild concerns. However, given that access to general BH therapy is limited, let alone access to specialty care and/or evidence-based treatments like CBT, PCPs are encouraged to use pharmacologic interventions alone, even for mild cases, if access to BH services is delayed or difficult. Following SSRIs, benzodiazepines are the second most common medication prescribed for ARDs in adolescents.[22] This is concerning as benzodiazepines are generally NOT recommended for ARD as the physiologic blunting of the fight, flight, freeze response is akin to an avoidance strategy that offers short-term relief but maintains and even worsens anxiety levels once it wears off as well as posing risk for dependence.[23]

Although PCPs are tasked with the difficult task of managing the mental health surge in youth, they often describe professional competency and time constraints in their ability to meet this need.[24] For consultation for pharmacologic treatment, PCPs are encouraged to utilize published treatment guidelines and consultative services such as Child Psychiatry Access Programs, such as the Telephonic Psychiatric Services (TiPS) in Pennsylvania, as a tool for PCPs to access real-time psychiatric support from CAPs.[25] In addition, the past few decades have seen an increase in integrated primary care (IPC) models where BH providers collaborate with PCPs and/or are colocated in PC practices. In fact, after outpatient and school settings, the third most common setting in which youth obtain BH therapeutic intervention is PC (10%).[15] The role of a BH provider in PC is multifaceted and includes assessment, consultation, case management, interfacing with schools, bridging care, and brief interventions. Given that anxiety concerns are the most common referral for BH providers in PC across all ages,[26] it is imperative that assessment and brief intervention for anxiety be integrated into PC practices. Despite exposure being the active ingredient in treatment for anxiety, studies have shown that compared to other interventions such as relaxation, exposure is infrequently used in IPC.[27] Given that consultation and/or intervention of anxiety in IPC is time-limited, it is recommended that providers prioritize psychoeducation of exposure frameworks to patients/caregivers, encourage approach behaviors toward feared situations, aid families in planning exposure practices at home, and help caregivers remove accommodations of anxious avoidance. Indeed, models of intervention for anxiety in PC that prioritize behavioral change through exposures, such as brief behavioral therapy, have showed positive effects for adolescents.[28] For both medical and BH providers in PC, it is recommended that psychoeducation about anxiety for patients and families be focused on the exposure framework rather than coping or relaxation skills, where families can be encouraged to start making behavioral changes that interfere with the growing avoidance cycle while waiting for therapy services. Given provider shortages and long wait times for specialty outpatient behavioral therapy, it is recommended that mild presentations of anxiety disorders be treated within PC when possible, especially given the escalating avoidance trajectories of untreated anxiety disorders, and referral to outpatient treatment settings be reserved for more moderate and severe presentations.

CLINICS CARE POINTS

- Particularly vulnerable populations for clinical anxiety post-quarantine include adolescent girls, minoritized populations, and those with LGBTQI identities and/or a history of trauma.
- It is important to carefully assess the extent to which anxiety "make sense" and is/was functionally relevant to one's surroundings.
- A blend of traditional CBT and third wave approaches incorporating values, acceptance, and distress tolerance is recommended. Exposures are favored for nonfunctional increases in anxiety (eg, social anxiety).
- In-person schooling is recommended, especially for anxious teens.
- A hybrid telehealth/in-person treatment model has the best potential to be effective in treatment of ARD.
- Decision making around proportion of telehealth versus in-person care for ARD should be collaboratively decided on by patients, caregivers, and clinicians based on cost/benefit analyses of access, engagement, and potential effectiveness.
- Given provider shortages and long wait lists, it is recommended that treatment for anxiety-related disorders also be provided outside of traditional outpatient settings such as schools and PC practices.
- PCPs are encouraged to manage medication for ARD, most commonly SSRIs, and reserve referral to CAPs for youth with severe presentations, complex mental health comorbidities and/or medical conditions, those that are failing SSRI trials in PC or experiencing side effects.
- PCPs are encouraged to seek out consultative services to aid in medication decision making including Child Psychiatry Access Programs, available in most states, such as the TiPS in Pennsylvania. Accessible through https://www.nncpap.org/
- PCPs are encouraged to obtain educational opportunities for ARD.
  - Pediatric Mental Health Minute: https://www.aap.org/en/patient-care/mental-health-minute/
  - The REACH Institute: https://thereachinstitute.org/

DISCLOSURE

Dr T.D. Benton is on the AFSP Board, Friends Central School Board, and Juvenile Law Center Board, serves as AACAP President, and recieves NIH/PCORI funding.

REFERENCES

1. Racine N, McArthur BA, Cooke JE, et al. Global Prevalence of Depressive and Anxiety Symptoms in Children and Adolescents During COVID-19: A Meta-analysis. JAMA Pediatr 2021;175(11):1142–50.
2. Madigan S, Racine N, Vaillancourt T, et al. Changes in Depression and Anxiety Among Children and Adolescents From Before to During the COVID-19 Pandemic: A Systematic Review and Meta-analysis. JAMA Pediatr 2023;177(6): 567–81.
3. Hawes MT, Szenczy AK, Olino TM, et al. Trajectories of depression, anxiety and pandemic experiences; A longitudinal study of youth in New York during the Spring-Summer of 2020. Psychiatr Res 2021;298:113778.
4. Salerno JP, Williams ND, Gattamorta KA. LGBTQ populations: Psychologically vulnerable communities in the COVID-19 pandemic. Psychol Trauma 2020; 12(S1):S239–42.
5. Strasser MA, Sumner PJ, Meyer D. COVID-19 news consumption and distress in young people: A systematic review. J Affect Disord 2022;300:481–91.
6. Mlawer F, Moore CC, Hubbard JA, et al. Pre-pandemic peer relations predict adolescents' internalizing response to Covid-19. Research on Child and Adolescent Psychopathology 2021;50(5):649–57.
7. Santibañez L., Guarino C.M., The effects of absenteeism on academic and social-emotional outcomes: Lessons for COVID-19, *Educational Researcher*, 50 (6), 2021, 392-400. https://doi.org/10.3102/0013189X21994488.
8. Krzyzaniak N, Greenwood H, Scott AM, et al. The effectiveness of telehealth versus face-to face interventions for anxiety disorders: A systematic review and meta-analysis. J Telemed Telecare 2021. https://doi.org/10.1177/1357633X211053738.
9. Islam S, Sanchez AL, McDermott CL, et al. To proceed via telehealth or not? considerations for pediatric anxiety and related disorders beyond COVID-19. Cognit Behav Pract 2023.
10. Mautone JA, Cabello B, Egan TE, et al. Exploring predictors of treatment engagement in urban integrated primary care. Clinical Practice in Pediatric Psychology 2020;8(3):228–40.
11. Mautone JA, Wolk CB, Cidav Z, et al. Strategic implementation planning for integrated behavioral health services in pediatric primary care. Implement Res Pract 2021. https://doi.org/10.1177/2633489520987558.
12. Kodjebacheva GD, Tang C, Groesbeck F, et al. Telehealth use in pediatric care during the COVID-19 pandemic: a qualitative study on the perspectives of caregivers. Children 2023;10(2):311.
13. Lu W, Todhunter-Reid A, Mitsdarffer ML, et al. Barriers and facilitators for mental health service use among racial/ethnic minority adolescents: a systematic review of literature. Front Public Health 2021;9:641605.
14. Chakawa A. Division of Developmental and Behavioral Health SoPP, Children's Mercy Hospitals and Clinics, Kansas City, MO, USA, University of Missouri Kansas City School of Medicine KC, MO, USA, et al. COVID-19, Telehealth, and Pediatric Integrated Primary Care: Disparities in Service Use. J Pediatr Psychol 2023;46(9):1063–75.

15. Duong MT, Bruns EJ, Lee K, et al. Rates of mental health service utilization by children and adolescents in schools and other common service settings: a systematic review and meta-analysis. Adm Pol Ment Health 2020;48(3):420–39.
16. Zhang Q, Wang J, Neitzel A. School-based mental health interventions targeting depression or anxiety: a meta-analysis of rigorous randomized controlled trials for school-aged children and adolescents. J Youth Adolesc 2022;52(1):195–217.
17. Njoroge WFM, Hostutler CA, Schwartz BS, et al. Integrated behavioral health in pediatric primary care. Curr Psychiatr Rep 2016;18(12):1–8.
18. Keares PP, Pho NT, Larson RS, et al. A comparison of pediatric mental health diagnoses and selective serotonin reuptake inhibitor prescribing before and during the COVID-19 pandemic. J Adolesc Health 2023;73(2).
19. Mental health toolkit | AAP toolkits. American Academy of Pediatrics; 2023. Available at: https://publications.aap.org/toolkits/pages/Mental-Health-Toolkit.
20. US Preventive Services Task Force, University of California LA. Screening for anxiety in children and adolescents: US preventive services task force recommendation statement. JAMA 2023;328(14):1438–44.
21. Walter HJ, Bukstein OG, Abright AR, et al. Clinical practice guideline for the assessment and treatment of children and adolescents with anxiety disorders. J Am Acad Child Adolesc Psychiatr 2020;59(10):1107–24.
22. Bushnell GA, Compton SN, Dusetzina SB, et al. Treating pediatric anxiety: Initial use of SSRIs and other anti-anxiety prescription medications. J Clin Psychiatr 2018;79(1).
23. Bandelow B, Sher L, Bunevicius R, et al. Guidelines for the pharmacological treatment of anxiety disorders, obsessive-compulsive disorder and posttraumatic stress disorder in primary care. Int J Psychiatr Clin Pract 2012;16(2).
24. Bettencourt AF, Ferro RA, Williams J-LL, et al. Pediatric primary care provider comfort with mental health practices: a needs assessment of regions with shortages of treatment access. Acad Psychiatr 2021;45(4):429–34.
25. Sullivan K, George P, Horowitz K. Addressing National workforce shortages by funding child psychiatry access programs. Pediatrics 2021;147(1):e20194012. https://doi.org/10.1542/peds.2019-4012.
26. Okoroji C, Mack Kolsky R, Williamson AA, et al. Integrated behavioral health in pediatric primary care: rates of consultation requests and treatment duration. Child Youth Care Forum 2023;1–16.
27. Blossom JB, Jungbluth N, Dillon-Naftolin E, et al. treatment for anxiety disorders in the pediatric primary care setting. Child Adolesc Psychiatr Clin N Am 2023; 32(3):601–11.
28. Schwartz KTG, Kado-Walton M, Dickerson JF, et al. Brief behavioral therapy for anxiety and depression in pediatric primary care: breadth of intervention impact. J Am Acad Child Adolesc Psychiatry 2023;62(2):230–43.

Post-Acute Sequelae of SARS-CoV-2 Infection and Its Impact on Adolescents and Young Adults

Check for updates

Camille A. Broussard, MD, MPH[a],*, Alba Azola, MD[b,c], Peter C. Rowe, MD[d]

KEYWORDS

- Long COVID • Post-COVID-19 condition
- Post-acute sequelae of SARS CoV-2 infection • Myalgic encephalomyelitis
- Chronic fatigue syndrome • Orthostatic intolerance • Adolescent

KEY POINTS

- Post-acute sequelae of SARS CoV-2 infection (PASC) in adolescents and young adults (AYAs) presents heterogeneously, often with multisystem involvement.
- Between 3 and 6 months after infection, the most common persistent symptoms reported are fever, sore throat, fatigue or muscle weakness, and sleep disturbances.
- A subset of AYAs with persistent symptoms 6 months post-acute SARS CoV-2 infection meet criteria for myalgic encephalomyelitis/chronic fatigue syndrome, among whom fatigue, cognitive difficulties, post-exertional malaise, sleep disturbance, and symptoms of orthostatic intolerance are most common.
- PASC can be incredibly debilitating for AYAs in physical, social, and emotional domains which may interrupt normal adolescent development and transition to adulthood.
- Primary care providers have a key role in initial diagnosis, assessment, and treatment for the numerous AYAs affected by PASC.

---

[a] Department of Pediatrics, Division of Adolescent & Young Adult Medicine, Johns Hopkins School of Medicine, 200 North Wolfe Street Room 2067, Baltimore, MD 21287, USA; [b] Department of Pediatrics, Division of Adolescent & Young Adult Medicine, Johns Hopkins School of Medicine, 200 North Wolfe Street Room 2069, Baltimore, MD 21287, USA; [c] Department of Physical Medicine and Rehabilitation, Johns Hopkins School of Medicine, 200 North Wolfe Street Room 2069, Baltimore, MD 21287, USA; [d] Department of Pediatrics, Division of Adolescent & Young Adult Medicine, Johns Hopkins School of Medicine, 200 North Wolfe Street Room 2077, Baltimore, MD 21287, USA
* Corresponding author.
E-mail address: camille.broussard@jhmi.edu

Pediatr Clin N Am 71 (2024) 613–630
https://doi.org/10.1016/j.pcl.2024.04.004   pediatric.theclinics.com

THE COMPLEXITY OF DEFINING POST-ACUTE SEQUELAE OF SARS-Cov-2 INFECTION

Discussions about what constitutes post-acute sequelae of SARS Cov-2 infection (PASC), also referred to as long COVID and post-COVID-19 condition, have been occurring within health care settings, research institutions, governments, communities, schools, families, media, and among patients. PASC has been identified in both adult and pediatric populations and varying definitions have been developed[1,2] (**Table 1**). The Centers for Disease Control and Prevention utilizes a time frame of symptoms lasting at least 4 weeks after acute COVID-19 infection, while the World Health Organization (WHO) utilizes a time frame of at least 2 months. The WHO includes a separate definition for children and adolescents.

Clinically, PASC has a heterogenous presentation with numerous phenotypes affecting multiple systems. No underlying pathophysiology or diagnostic biomarker has been identified; however, hypothesized pathophysiologic mechanisms include immune dysregulation, microbiota dysbiosis, autoimmunity, and endothelial and neurologic dysfunction.[3] Most research on PASC has been focused on adult populations. In this article, the authors discuss available knowledge on PASC in adolescents and young adults (AYAs), a group that encompasses ages 12 to 25 years.

BURDEN AND IMPACT OF POST-ACUTE SEQUELAE OF SARS Cov-2 INFECTION ON ADOLESCENTS AND YOUNG ADULTS

Although there are reports of milder COVID-19 disease and lower hospitalization rates in the pediatric population,[4] AYAs are still at risk for developing PASC. Published prevalence estimates vary widely, ranging from 4% to 25%, in part due to varying case definitions.[5–8] Adolescents are typically included in aggregate pediatric data, while young adults are typically included in aggregate adult data. However, AYAs are a unique group with unique needs. Obtaining an appropriate control group not previously infected with COVID-19 to accurately compare PASC prevalence rates and the impact of PASC on the AYA population is challenging. Thus, the true number of AYAs that have or will be affected by PASC is largely unknown. Additionally, there are few specialty PASC clinics, typically limited to urban areas, most focused on the adult population, and without a sufficient number of providers to see all patients. Thus, it is imperative that primary care providers become more comfortable in the recognition, assessment, and initial management of AYAs with PASC.

Impact on Functioning

Given the complex and multisystemic nature of PASC, the effects on AYAs are widespread, with variability in symptom severity for each individual. This includes impacts on physical, social, and emotional functioning. Importantly for AYAs, the impact on normal adolescent and young adulthood development is critical to examine. AYAs during this period of life should be developing their identity, engaging in social activities, and transitioning to adulthood. However, many AYAs with PASC cannot engage in these developmental milestones due to the severity of their illness. Profound fatigue may physically limit social activities as well as activities of daily living. This fatigue along with post-exertional malaise (PEM) and respiratory difficulties may limit engagement in sports or other extracurricular activities that are a large part of adolescent identity.[9] School absences have also increased in those with PASC, detrimentally impacting educational and career attainment.[9,10] Furthermore, the brain fog and concentration difficulties may also limit the ability of AYAs to engage in schoolwork and/or work responsibilities. Without the ability to achieve further educational progress or engage in the workforce due to severe PASC illness, AYAs may need to rely on adult

Table 1
Definitions of post-acute sequelae of SARS CoV-2 infection

	Centers for Disease Control and Prevention	World Health Organization[1]
Definition	Working definition (as of July 20, 2023) Broadly defined as signs, symptoms, and conditions that continue or develop after acute COVID-19 infection. Symptoms: • Present 4 weeks or more after the initial phase of infection • May be multisystemic • May present with a relapsing—remitting pattern and progression or worsening over time, with the possibility of severe and life-threatening events even months or years after infection	Consensus definition (as of February 16, 2023) Occurs in individuals with a history of confirmed or probable SARS-CoV-2 infection. Symptoms: • Lasting at least 2 mo which initially occurred within 3 mo of acute COVID-19 • Impact everyday functioning • May be new onset following initial recovery or persist from the initial illness • May fluctuate or relapse
Specifics for pediatric population	No pediatric/adolescent-specific definition	Fatigue, altered smell/anosmia, and *anxiety* may be symptoms more frequently reported in children and adolescents. Functioning domains to consider: • Eating habits • Physical activity • Behavior • Academic performance • Social functions (interactions with friends, peers, family) • Developmental milestones

caregivers and/or assess options for disability status. Recently, guidance on PASC eligibility for classification as a disability under the Americans with Disabilities Act was developed.[11] Finally, having a profound interruption in health and well-being for AYAs may lead to secondary depression and/or anxiety. It is important to note that the neuropsychiatric sequelae of SARS CoV-2 infection on AYAs must be investigated independently from the mental health impact of the general COVID-19 pandemic in this population. Studies to date do not disentangle the experience of the pandemic with the impact of having PASC-related neuropsychiatric condition.

Prognosis

Long-term prognosis for AYAs with PASC is still an area of active investigation and is largely unknown. Observational studies following AYAs longitudinally suggest that patients who do not recover by 6 to 9 months have a lower probability of recovering within 1 to 2 years.[12] A similar investigation into recovery among adults with PASC revealed less than 10% of patients fully recovered and those that did recover were more likely to be less symptomatic.[13] If AYAs with PASC that additionally meet criteria for myalgic encephalomyelitis/chronic fatigue syndrome (ME/CFS) follow prognosis trends for those with ME/CFS pre-COVID-19, we may expect recovery (returning back to pre-illness level of functioning) or improvement to take 2 to 5 years, and a subset of patients who will continue to experience disabling symptoms for more than 10 years.[14,15] However, consensus on the assessment of recovery specific to AYAs has not yet been established.[16,17] A core set of 11 health outcomes that should be measured in adults has been developed by consensus and a pediatric version is in development.[18] This will allow for better harmonization of data and to have more meaningful health outcomes to follow for affected patients.

SYMPTOM PROFILES

AYAs with PASC have presented heterogeneously with a variety of symptoms; some presenting with one persistent symptom and some presenting with multiple persistent symptoms (**Table 2**).[3,19–22] Fatigue, concentration difficulties, and PEM (when patients experience a "crash" or exacerbation of symptoms lasting more than 24 hours after physical, cognitive, or orthostatic stress) are 3 of the most common symptoms reported by AYAs with PASC.[5,8,12,20,23,24] Respiratory symptoms are more frequently reported in the initial weeks to 3 months after acute infection[25]; however, pulmonary function tests are rarely impaired in children and adolescents except for those with history of severe COVID-19 infection.[26] Anosmia and ageusia/dysgeusia have also been found to be quite common in pediatric PASC and appear to gradually improve over time.[27,28] Thus, providers must have a high index of suspicion when AYAs with a history of past COVID-19 present with a variety of symptoms that otherwise cannot be explained by another diagnosis.

Additionally, research in adult populations with PASC has identified 4 symptom profile clusters.[29] These include subgroups primarily experiencing (1) loss of or change in smell or taste; (2) PEM and fatigue; (3) brain fog, PEM, and fatigue; and (4) fatigue, PEM, dizziness, brain fog, gastrointestinal (GI), and palpitations. Similar explorations are underway in adolescent populations. Identification of symptom profile clusters may aid in more targeted management based on phenotype.

Orthostatic Intolerance in PASC

Orthostatic intolerance (OI) in general and postural orthostatic tachycardia syndrome (POTS) specifically are being recognized as common contributors to PASC in

Table 2
Common symptoms in adolescents and young adults with post-acute sequelae of SARS CoV-2 infection by system

Body System	Symptoms
Systemic/constitutional	• Dizziness • Lightheadedness • Fatigue • Post-exertional malaise • Exercise intolerance • Brain fog/concentration difficulties • Sleep disturbances • Menstrual irregularities
Neuropsychiatric	• Headache • Peripheral neuropathy • Anxiety • Depression
Otolaryngologic	• Anosmia • Ageusia/dysgeusia • Dysphagia • Dysphonia • Nasal congestion • Sore throat
Cardiovascular	• Palpitations • Chest pain • Tachycardia • Syncope
Pulmonary	• Cough • Dyspnea
Gastrointestinal	• Abdominal pain • Nausea • Bowel irregularities • Lack of appetite
Musculoskeletal	• Myalgias • Arthralgias • Muscle weakness

AYAs[20,30–32] as has been reported extensively in adults.[33–37] Some AYAs who undergo testing for autonomic dysfunction via a 10 min passive standing test do not meet formal criteria for POTS, but have chronic orthostatic symptoms.[31,38] In adults, individuals with similar symptom profiles associated with a normal heart rate and blood pressure response to orthostatic stress nonetheless develop a mean 24% reduction in cerebral blood flow compared to supine values (vs a mean 7% reduction in healthy controls).[39] Thus, despite normal heart rate and blood pressure responses, many, if not all, of these individuals warrant trials of therapy directed at OI. Furthermore, COVID-19 infection can worsen pre-existing OI symptoms or OI can develop for the first time in AYAs post-COVID-19.

Symptoms of ME/CFS

Finally, a subset of AYAs have persistent and debilitating symptoms beyond 6 months and meet the Institute of Medicine criteria for ME/CFS.[20,30,32,40] COVID-19 infection joins other infectious triggers for ME/CFS, including commonly Epstein–Barr virus (EBV).[41] While the main risk factor for ME/CFS 6 months after EBV infection is the severity of the infection,[41] the severity of symptoms and impaired function following SARS-CoV-2 infection can be independent of the degree of initial illness and can follow milder asymptomatic infection for non-hospitalized patients.[12,42] Criteria for diagnosing ME/CFS post-COVID-19 infection include (1) substantial impairment in the ability to engage in pre-illness levels of activity that lasts for more than 6 months and is accompanied by profound fatigue not substantially alleviated by rest; (2) PEM; (3) unrefreshing sleep; and either (4a) cognitive dysfunction ("brain fog") or (4b) OI.[43] These symptoms should be present at least half the time, and with at least moderate severity. The focus for the assessment and management strategies in this article will focus largely on this subset of AYAs with ME/CFS after COVID-19 infection.

RISK AND PROTECTIVE FACTORS FOR POST-ACUTE SEQUELAE OF SARS CoV-2 INFECTION

Risk factors for PASC identified through observational studies include having pre-existing comorbidities, assigned female sex at birth, age older than 10 years, and hospitalization or severe illness or during acute COVID-19 infection.[6,7,12,25,44] Comorbid conditions that confer an increased risk include allergic disease, asthma, obesity, anxiety, heart disease, and neurologic diseases.[12,44] Additionally, pediatric patients who reported anosmia and/or dysgeusia during acute COVID-19 infection and those infected with a pre-Omicron variant appear to have a higher risk of persistent anosmia and dysgeusia.[27] In the adult PASC literature, reinfection with COVID-19 appears to be associated with an increased risk for PASC.[45]

Observational studies in adults suggest that vaccination against COVID-19 may protect against PASC[46]; small pediatric studies suggest a similar trend.[6] One study among older adults showed that treatment with Paxlovid within 5 days of a positive test for those with at least one risk factor for severe COVID-19 was associated with a reduced risk of PASC.[47] Studies with larger sample sizes will be needed to confirm whether these confer a statistically significant degree of protection for AYAs.

ASSESSMENT AND MANAGEMENT STRATEGIES
Assessment of Symptoms Suggestive of Post-Acute Sequelae of SARS CoV-2 Infection

AYAs typically present to primary care with symptoms as discussed earlier (for case example, see **Box 1**). While this can present quite a challenge for primary care providers and various subspecialty providers to whom patients are often referred, some models of care have been developed.[48–50] Additionally, there is a consensus guidance statement regarding the assessment and treatment of PASC in children and adolescents that details a system-based approach.[20] For young adults, there are additional consensus adult guidelines for the assessment and treatment of PASC-related fatigue and autonomic dysfunction that providers can reference, as these are some of the most common presenting symptoms.[51,52]

In general, the first task is to obtain a symptom inventory and to assess the functional impact of PASC symptoms on activities of daily living, schooling, and vocational and extracurricular/social activities. In time-limited primary care visits, providers can develop a triage list of the most important symptoms to manage first. Symptoms might be triaged into higher priority levels based on the most debilitating symptoms, most treatable symptoms, need for subspecialty referral, or patient-driven.[53] Subsequently, early screening for PEM and OI (with an in-office 10 min passive standing test—see **Fig. 1** for example form)[54,55] is recommended, especially given the elevated prevalence and treatable nature of OI in PASC. Finally, a treatment plan may be developed

---

Box 1
Case example

A 15 year old previously healthy female presents for evaluation of multiple symptoms including fatigue, dizziness, palpitations, shortness of breath, abdominal pain, diarrhea, vomiting, facial flushing, hot/cold intolerance, and brain fog. Symptoms emerged after COVID-19 infection. During the acute infection her resting heart rate was between 150 and 160 beats per minute (bpm); she experienced extreme fatigue along with cough and nasal congestion. Acute respiratory symptoms resolved after 1 month but presenting symptoms have persisted for more than 9 months. She is sleeping 8 to 10 hours nightly but awakens unrefreshed. She requires 1 to 2 days of recovery after an active day. She can no longer engage in sports and has difficulty with attention in class. This has severely affected quality of life. Hot showers bother her now with lightheadedness in the shower with a need to shower sitting down. Family history is notable for an older sister with hypermobile type Ehlers–Danlos Syndrome and ME/CFS.

On examination, facial flushing was present. Heart rate 105 while sitting. Mild tenderness to palpation in epigastric region. Diffuse striae present on upper arms, back, abdomen, hips, and behind knees (body mass index 23). Beighton score was 0/9. She developed arm fatigue within 20 seconds and palpitations at 55 seconds during an abbreviated 60 s elevated arm stress test. An in-office passive 10 min standing test revealed a 61 bpm increase in heart rate from lowest supine to peak standing value along with report of fatigue, dizziness, brain fog, and palpitations.

The patient met criteria for ME/CFS post-COVID-19 infection. History, symptoms, and examination were also consistent with the following ME/CFS co-morbid conditions: POTS, facial flushing suggestive of MCAS, problems with GI motility, TOS symptoms, and secondary depression. Symptomatic treatment for each co-morbid condition was initiated. Allergies, facial flushing, and GI issues improved with levocetirizine and famotidine. Unfortunately, trials of methylphenidate, selective serotonin reuptake inhibitor, and a beta blocker have not controlled POTS symptoms. Overall, the patient has persistent symptoms, now 21 months post-COVID-19 infection.

---

based on this initial assessment, although providers should be flexible with treatment plans as PASC symptoms may evolve over time.

For AYAs presenting with PASC symptoms greater than 6 months, we recommend having a structured approach (**Fig. 2**) to identify those that meet criteria for ME/CFS and to assess for common comorbidities of ME/CFS (**Fig. 3** and **Table 3**). These comorbidities originally studied in and associated with ME/CFS have begun to also appear as comorbidities with PASC. Common shared comorbidities include headaches,[56–59] OI,[30,60–62] mast cell activation syndrome (MCAS),[63] and joint hypermobility with associated pain conditions.[64–66] The other comorbidities around the multidisciplinary wheel in **Fig. 3** have been associated with ME/CFS and OI in AYAs in previous literature[67–71]; however, further investigation is needed to assess whether all the comorbidities are also associated with PASC. Additionally, we recommend screening for depression (eg, Beck Depression Inventory II, PHQ-9 Modified for Teens) and cognitive dysfunction (eg, PedsQL Multidimensional Fatigue Scale) as these problems may not be apparent within a single encounter.

Management Strategies

Treatment of PASC for those that meet ME/CFS criteria includes symptomatic management of identified comorbidities that are common in ME/CFS (**Table 4**).[3,72] Treatment should be individualized to the patient's presenting symptoms using typical treatments. However, it is important to note that symptoms of OI are among the most treatable symptoms of PASC. Management of OI begins with modification of environmental triggers that provoke symptoms (eg, prolonged standing, warm

	Blood Pressure	Heart Rate	FTG	LH	COG	HA	Other
10 Minute Office Passive Standing Test							
Patient Name: _____							
SUPINE							
1 min							
2 min							
3 min							
4 min							
5 min							
STANDING							
1 min							
2 min							
3 min							
4 min							
5 min							
6 min							
7 min							
8 min							
9 min							
10 min							
SUPINE							
1 min							
2 min							

Acrocyanosis observed during test: ( ) No   ( ) Yes, mild   ( ) Yes, moderate to severe

Fig. 1. In-office 10 min passive standing test form to assess for orthostatic intolerance. *Instructions: Lie the patient supine on examination table with automated blood pressure cuff placed on right upper arm (recording blood pressure [BP] and heart rate [HR] at 1 min intervals throughout the test). After 5 minutes of lying supine, the patient stands with heels 2 to 6 inches away from the wall and upper back leaning against the wall. The patient remains standing in this position for 10 minutes. The test can be stopped early at patient request or in the event of severe presyncope symptoms—the patient should be instructed to sit or lie down if this occurs. After 10 minutes upright, the patient returns to the supine position for an additional 2 minutes of BP and HR recording. Ask patients about intensity of orthostatic symptoms on a 0 to 10 scale (0 being none, 10 being the worst) after BPs and HRs are recorded. Movement (especially while standing) and conversation throughout the test should be kept to a minimum. See Appendix G in reference*[38] *for more detailed information for this test.* ACRO, acrocyanosis; COG, Brain fog; FTG, Fatigue; HA, Headache; HOT, Warmth/hot flash; LH, Lightheadedness/dizziness; NAU, Nausea; PN, Muscle pain/ache; SOB, trouble breathing; SW, Sweating.

environments), along with the non-pharmacologic measures described in **Table 4**. Most individuals with clinically significant OI will also benefit from pharmacologic treatments (described in more detail in references[30,38]). Aggressively managing OI may bring profound symptomatic improvements for AYAs with PASC, as OI negatively impacts level of fatigue, activity intolerance, cognitive dysfunction, and other comorbidities on the multidisciplinary wheel. The most common subspecialty referrals from

Detailed history	Physical exam	Labs & Procedures
• Onset & duration • Typical functioning & impact on life • Assessing for post-exertional malaise • Assessing for orthostatic intolerance • Assessing for cognitive dysfunction • Assessing for associated conditions	• General exam • Neurologic exam • Beighton scoring assessing for joint hypermobility • Range of motion evaluation assessing for restrictions	• CBC, CMP, thyroid studies, ESR/CRP, iron panel, vitamin B12, vitamin D, Celiac disease screening, urinalysis, histamine/tryptase • Orthostatic testing with 10-minute passive standing test

Fig. 2. Structured approach to assessing patients presenting with post-acute sequelae of SARS CoV-2 infection symptoms concerning for myalgic encephalomyelitis/chronic fatigue syndrome.

primary care providers for patients with PASC include physical medicine and rehabilitation, neurology, pulmonology, cardiology, and physical therapy.[73,74] Finally, management strategies that have been proposed are based on expert and consensus guidance. Thus, more research is needed to elucidate the best evidence-based strategies for continued improvement in functioning and quality of life for AYAs with PASC.

Assessing for clinically significant or patient-identified improvement in either symptom, functioning, or quality of life is critical when caring for AYAs with PASC. We recommend utilizing questionnaires at initial evaluation and again periodically throughout care. Examples of questionnaires that can be used to track health-related quality of life over time include Pediatric Quality of Life Inventory (PedsQL) 4.0 Generic Core,[75] PedsQL 3.0 Multidimensional Fatigue Scale,[76] and the EQ-5D.[77]

Recommendations for Pacing to Avoid Post-Exertional Malaise

Providers should recommend AYAs with PASC engage in pacing to avoid PEM by adjusting their activity level within the limits imposed by their illness.[78] Similarly, pacing has been utilized in fatigue management in ME/CFS populations.[79] Pacing suggests

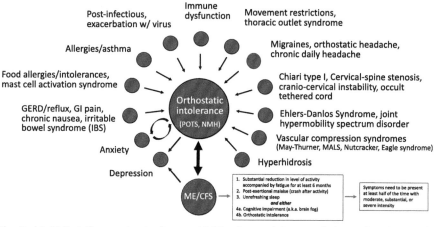

Fig. 3. Multidisciplinary wheel of comorbidities in myalgic encephalomyelitis/chronic fatigue syndrome.

Table 3
Review of symptoms for common comorbidities in myalgic encephalomyelitis/chronic fatigue syndrome post-COVID-19 infection

Comorbidity	ROS Questions
Orthostatic intolerance	• Lightheaded or unwell after 5 min of standing • Worse with hot weather, hot shower, standing in line/shopping, walking in mall, menses • Any salt craving
Mast cell activation syndrome	• Hives • Facial flushing or body erythema • Unexplained rashes • Exaggerated reaction to insect bites/stings • New onset food/medication sensitivities
Milk protein intolerance	• Epigastric abdominal pain • Early satiety • Reflux symptoms • Frequent mouth ulcers • Feel unwell 2–4 h after diary intake
Thoracic outlet syndrome	• Arm paresthesia, arm fatigue, or general fatigue with arms overhead or extended (eg, driving, reaching up for object, shampooing hair) • Trapezius or shoulder discomfort/pain
Joint hypermobility	• Double jointed • Tricks with limbs (eg, able to put leg behind head) • Dislocations/subluxations • Active in dancing, cheerleading, gymnastics, and/or swimming

breaking activity tasks into smaller chunks, switching between activities that require different muscle groups (eg, reading vs walking), resting briefly between activities, and gradually increasing activity to avoid a relapse of symptoms. The key advice is to avoid both underexertion and overexertion. Adequately treating OI is often a prerequisite to tolerating increased activity, but once autonomic function improves, patients can gradually increase activity on their own without provoking PEM.[38] Additionally, our clinical experience has been that gentle manual physical therapy to address movement restrictions and neuromuscular tightness/strain may help a patient to tolerate other types of exercise. Pacing might be challenging for AYAs who were accustomed to engaging in sports activity before becoming ill. Based on experience in ME/CFS care, strict, structured, or graded exercise protocols may be harmful as this can worsen PEM and PASC symptoms and should not be recommended for those AYAs meeting ME/CFS criteria.[3] Finally, providers can offer a combination of face-to-face and telemedicine visits based on patient ability which supports pacing as some patients will experience PEM after face-to-face visits.

SUPPORT FOR ADOLESCENTS AND YOUNG ADULTS WITH POST-ACUTE SEQUELAE OF SARS CoV-2 INFECTION

Given the impact of PASC symptoms on school/work attendance and performance, school and/or work accommodations can be beneficial for most AYAs with PASC. Examples of academic accommodations and sample letters written to schools can be found in Appendices D and E in reference[38]. These can include

• A later start to the day as mornings can be more difficult symptom-wise.
• Flexibility in assignment due dates and scheduling of testing dates.

Table 4
Potential directed therapies for common comorbid conditions in post-acute sequelae of SARS CoV-2 infection

Common Comorbid Condition	Potential Directed Therapies

Orthostatic Intolerance	• Non-pharmacologic: 2–3 L of hydration daily, increased dietary salt intake/salt tablets/electrolyte supplements, compression garments, cooling garments, postural counter-maneuvers.
	• Vasoconstrictors
	  • Midodrine 5–10 mg TID, methylphenidate/dextroamphetamine, SSRI/SNRI
	• Volume expanders
	  • Fludrocortisone 0.1 mg daily, clonidine 0.1 mg daily, combined contraceptives, desmopressin
	• Decrease heart rate/catecholamine release or effect
	  • Beta-blocker, pyridostigmine bromide 30–60 mg BID to TID, ivabradine 2.5–7.5 mg BID

Mast Cell Activation Syndrome	Famotidine 40 mg QD to BID, oral cromolyn 200 mg QID, Nasalcrom OTC, loratadine/cetirizine/fexofenadine, montelukast 5–10 mg QHS, quercetin 500–1000 mg BID
Chronic pain	Low dose naltrexone 0.5–4.5 mg daily, gabapentin, pregabalin, duloxetine, amitriptyline/nortripyline, finger ring splints for those with joint hypermobility of the fingers, joint stabilization sleeves
Milk protein intolerance	Dairy-free diet trial for at least 2 wk
Thoracic outlet syndrome (TOS) and movement restrictions	Injection with analgesic or botulinum toxin in scalene muscles for TOS, manual physical therapy

- Extended time for test-taking or ability to take breaks during tests.
- Flexibility with make-up work assignments and absences.

Given the lack of information on PASC, many patients have sought support via online platforms and social media-based online support groups. Providers can support patients by asking about potential support groups and ensuring that patients feel validated and safe to disclose their symptoms and how these symptoms are affecting quality of life and functioning.[53,80] Patients often also report difficulty navigating the health care system to obtain a diagnosis. Referrals for psychotherapy focused on coping with the new physical and mental impairments may be beneficial. Loss of function and decreased quality of life can contribute to development of new onset depression and anxiety symptoms or exacerbation of preexisting mental health conditions.

EQUITY IN CARING FOR ADOLESCENTS AND YOUNG ADULTS WITH POST-ACUTE SEQUELAE OF SARS CoV-2 INFECTION

Overwhelmingly, access to care for PASC has been limited to those who can navigate health care systems, afford to travel for care, afford off-label treatment, and/or have social capital to gain access to specialty clinics or knowledgeable providers. Reports in the media and medical literature call attention to PASC care being limited to mostly affluent, female, and White populations.[73,81–83] It is possible to improve access to care for racially, ethnically, and socioeconomically diverse patient populations living with PASC. Recent examples include the COVID-19 Recovery and Engagement Clinics in the Bronx, New York,[84] UT Health San Antonio Program,[48] the Northwestern Medicine Comprehensive COVID-19 Center,[74] and the ClinSeqSer[85] study in New Orleans,

Louisiana. Additionally, the US National Institutes of Health's RECOVER Initiative and reports from the Veterans Affairs databases[86] have reported more representative samples. Strategies have included partnering with community-based organizations, having case managers that understand the community, having providers with experience navigating Medicaid/Medicare, allowing self-referrals into clinics instead of solely physician-referral based models, and targeted outreach in underserved communities. A similar experience for the pediatric/adolescent population has not been described to our knowledge except for enrollment in the RECOVER Initiative pediatric cohort.[87] In order to reduce health inequities related to PASC in AYAs as well as prevent further widening of existing health disparities, we must be intentional about identifying and reducing barriers to care to increase access. We encourage PASC clinics to adopt an equity framework for access to care and learn from those examples that are making access more equitable.[88,89]

Primary care providers are also crucial in the goal of expanding access so that more patients can be seen near their home. Increasing primary care to subspecialty collaboration may assist with these endeavors and reducing referral bias from primary care to subspecialists is important.[90] Providing telemedicine appointments may also be an avenue to increasing access within primary care settings for patients who do not live near large academic centers. Thus, the education of primary care providers on recognition, assessment, and management of PASC is paramount.

SUMMARY

There still is much to be discovered regarding PASC in AYAs. Acute respiratory symptoms and problems with taste and smell generally improve within 1 to 5 months after infection. Common persistent symptoms after COVID-19 infection in AYAs include fatigue, cognitive difficulties, PEM, headaches, and lightheadedness. A subset of AYAs develop more substantial impairments in function similar to those seen in ME/CFS. As we await data from observational and interventional studies in PASC, many of the management strategies used for existing conditions like ME/CFS, OI, and MCAS can be applied to improve function and quality of life in AYAs with PASC(see **Box 1**).

CLINICS CARE POINTS

- Providers should highly suspect a diagnosis of PASC for AYAs presenting for care with multisystem symptoms after COVID-19 infection.

- Barriers in access to health care and other equity considerations limit PASC diagnosis in minoritized racial/ethnic groups, efforts for equitable care of people with PASC must be prioritized. Providers should conduct a comprehensive history, including assessment of level of function, physical examination, and screen for OI and PES to triage symptoms, initiate treatment, and facilitate subspecialty referrals for AYAs presenting with PASC symptoms.

- Providers can assess OI using an in-office 10 min passive standing test, monitoring for symptom provocation and changes in heart rate and blood pressure.

- Although there is no single therapy effective for all AYAs with PASC, many of the presenting symptoms are responsive to existing treatments for allergic inflammation, MCAS, OI, headaches, dysmenorrhea, depression/anxiety, or problems with attention.

DISCLOSURE

The authors have nothing to disclose.

REFERENCES

1. World Health Organization. A clinical case definition for post-COVID-19 condition in children and adolescents by expert consensus. 2023. Available at: https://www.who.int/publications/i/item/WHO-2019-nCoV-Post-COVID-19-condition-CA-Clinical-case-definition-2023-1. [Accessed 8 September 2023].
2. Centers for Disease Control and Prevention. Long COVID or Post-COVID Conditions. 2023. Available at: https://www.cdc.gov/coronavirus/2019-ncov/long-term-effects/index.html#:~:text=People%20call%20Long%20COVID%20by,of%20COVID%2C%20and%20chronic%20COVID. [Accessed 8 September 2023].
3. Davis HE, McCorkell L, Vogel JM, et al. Long COVID: major findings, mechanisms and recommendations. Nat Rev Microbiol 2023;21(3):133–46.
4. Zimmermann P, Curtis N. Coronavirus Infections in Children Including COVID-19: An Overview of the Epidemiology, Clinical Features, Diagnosis, Treatment and Prevention Options in Children. Pediatr Infect Dis J 2020;39(5):355–68.
5. Izquierdo-Pujol J, Moron-Lopez S, Dalmau J, et al. Post-COVID-19 Condition in Children and Adolescents: An Emerging Problem. Front Pediatr 2022;10:894204.
6. Morello R, Mariani F, Mastrantoni L, et al. Risk factors for post-COVID-19 condition (Long Covid) in children: a prospective cohort study. EClinicalMedicine 2023;59:101961.
7. Zheng YB, Zeng N, Yuan K, et al. Prevalence and risk factor for long COVID in children and adolescents: A meta-analysis and systematic review. J Infect Public Health 2023;16(5):660–72.
8. Lopez-Leon S, Wegman-Ostrosky T, Ayuzo del Valle NC, et al. Long-COVID in children and adolescents: a systematic review and meta-analyses. Sci Rep 2022;12:9950.
9. Gonzalez-Aumatell A, Bovo MV, Carreras-Abad C, et al. Social, Academic, and Health Status Impact of Long COVID on Children and Young People: An Observational, Descriptive, and Longitudinal Cohort Study. Child Basel Switz 2022;9(11):1677.
10. Kikkenborg Berg S, Dam Nielsen S, Nygaard U, et al. Long COVID symptoms in SARS-CoV-2-positive adolescents and matched controls (LongCOVIDKidsDK): a national, cross-sectional study. Lancet Child Adolesc Health 2022;6(4):240–8.
11. US Department of Health and Human Services. Guidance on "Long COVID" as a Disability Under the ADA, Section 504, and Section 1557. Available at: https://www.hhs.gov/civil-rights/for-providers/civil-rights-covid19/guidance-long-covid-disability/index.html#footnote10_0ac8mdc. [Accessed 8 September 2023].
12. Buonsenso D, Pazukhina E, Gentili C, et al. The Prevalence, Characteristics and Risk Factors of Persistent Symptoms in Non-Hospitalized and Hospitalized Children with SARS-CoV-2 Infection Followed-Up for up to 12 Months: A Prospective, Cohort Study in Rome, Italy. J Clin Med 2022;11(22):6772.
13. Mateu L, Tebe C, Loste C, et al. Determinants of the onset and prognosis of the post-COVID-19 condition: a 2-year prospective observational cohort study. Lancet Reg Health – Eur 2023;0(0). https://doi.org/10.1016/j.lanepe.2023.100724.
14. Rowe KS. Long Term Follow up of Young People With Chronic Fatigue Syndrome Attending a Pediatric Outpatient Service. Front Pediatr 2019;7:21.
15. van Geelen SM, Bakker RJ, Kuis W, et al. Adolescent Chronic Fatigue Syndrome: A Follow-up Study. Arch Pediatr Adolesc Med 2010;164(9):810–4.
16. Munblit D, Buonsenso D, Sigfrid L, et al. Post-COVID-19 condition in children: a COS is urgently needed. Lancet Respir Med 2022;10(7):628–9.

17. Munblit D, Sigfrid L, Warner JO. Setting Priorities to Address Research Gaps in Long-term COVID-19 Outcomes in Children. JAMA Pediatr 2021;175(11):1095–6.
18. Munblit D, Nicholson T, Akrami A, et al. A core outcome set for post-COVID-19 condition in adults for use in clinical practice and research: an international Delphi consensus study. Lancet Respir Med 2022;10(7):715–24.
19. Thallapureddy K, Thallapureddy K, Zerda E, et al. Long-Term Complications of COVID-19 Infection in Adolescents and Children. Curr Pediatr Rep 2022; 10(1):11–7.
20. Malone LA, Morrow A, Chen Y, et al. Multi-disciplinary collaborative consensus guidance statement on the assessment and treatment of post-acute sequelae of SARS-CoV-2 infection (PASC) in children and adolescents. PM&R 2022; 14(10):1241–69.
21. Chen EY, Burton JM, Johnston A, et al. Considerations in Children and Adolescents Related to Coronavirus Disease 2019 (COVID-19). Phys Med Rehabil Clin 2023. https://doi.org/10.1016/j.pmr.2023.03.004.
22. Jiang L, Li X, Nie J, et al. A Systematic Review of Persistent Clinical Features After SARS-CoV-2 in the Pediatric Population. Pediatrics 2023;152(2). e2022060351.
23. Fainardi V, Meoli A, Chiopris G, et al. Long COVID in Children and Adolescents. Life 2022;12(2):285.
24. Roessler M, Tesch F, Batram M, et al. Post-COVID-19-associated morbidity in children, adolescents, and adults: A matched cohort study including more than 157,000 individuals with COVID-19 in Germany. PLoS Med 2022;19(11):e1004122.
25. Baptista de Lima J, Salazar L, Fernandes A, et al. Long COVID in Children and Adolescents: A Retrospective Study in a Pediatric Cohort. Pediatr Infect Dis J 2023;42(4):e109–11.
26. Knoke L, Schlegtendal A, Maier C, et al. Pulmonary Function and Long-Term Respiratory Symptoms in Children and Adolescents After COVID-19. Front Pediatr 2022;10:851008.
27. Mariani F, Morello R, Traini DO, et al. Risk Factors for Persistent Anosmia and Dysgeusia in Children with SARS-CoV-2 Infection: A Retrospective Study. Children 2023;10(3):597.
28. Hahn LM, Manny E, Mamede F, et al. Post-COVID-19 Condition in Children. JAMA Pediatr 2023;e233239.
29. Thaweethai T, Jolley SE, Karlson EW, et al. Development of a Definition of Postacute Sequelae of SARS-CoV-2 Infection. JAMA 2023;329(22):1934–46.
30. Morrow AK, Malone LA, Kokorelis C, et al. Long-Term COVID 19 Sequelae in Adolescents: the Overlap with Orthostatic Intolerance and ME/CFS. Curr Pediatr Rep 2022;10(2):31–44.
31. Drogalis-Kim D, Kramer C, Duran S. Ongoing Dizziness Following Acute COVID-19 Infection: A Single Center Pediatric Case Series. Pediatrics 2022;150(2). e2022056860.
32. Petracek LS, Suskauer SJ, Vickers RF, et al. Adolescent and Young Adult ME/CFS After Confirmed or Probable COVID-19. Front Med 2021;8:668944.
33. Blitshteyn S, Whitelaw S. Postural orthostatic tachycardia syndrome (POTS) and other autonomic disorders after COVID-19 infection: a case series of 20 patients. Immunol Res 2021;69(2):205–11.
34. Dani M, Dirksen A, Taraborrelli P, et al. Autonomic dysfunction in "long COVID": rationale, physiology and management strategies. Clin Med Lond Engl 2021; 21(1):e63–7.

35. Hira R, Baker JR, Siddiqui T, et al. Objective Hemodynamic Cardiovascular Autonomic Abnormalities in Post-Acute Sequelae of COVID-19. Can J Cardiol 2023; 39(6):767–75.
36. Shouman K, Vanichkachorn G, Cheshire WP, et al. Autonomic dysfunction following COVID-19 infection: an early experience. Clin Auton Res Off J Clin Auton Res Soc 2021;31(3):385–94.
37. Miglis MG, Prieto T, Shaik R, et al. A case report of postural tachycardia syndrome after COVID-19. Clin Auton Res Off J Clin Auton Res Soc 2020;30(5): 449–51.
38. Rowe PC, Underhill RA, Friedman KJ, et al. Myalgic Encephalomyelitis/Chronic Fatigue Syndrome Diagnosis and Management in Young People: A Primer. Front Pediatr 2017;5:121.
39. van Campen C, Linda MC, Verheugt FWA, et al. Cerebral blood flow is reduced in ME/CFS during head-up tilt testing even in the absence of hypotension or tachycardia: A quantitative, controlled study using Doppler echography. Clin Neurophysiol Pract 2020;5:50–8.
40. Siberry VGR, Rowe PC. Pediatric Long COVID and Myalgic Encephalomyelitis/ Chronic Fatigue Syndrome. Pediatr Infect Dis J 2022;41(4):e139–41.
41. Katz BZ, Shiraishi Y, Mears CJ, et al. Chronic fatigue syndrome after infectious mononucleosis in adolescents. Pediatrics 2009;124(1):189–93.
42. Subramanian A, Nirantharakumar K, Hughes S, et al. Symptoms and risk factors for long COVID in non-hospitalized adults. Nat Med 2022;28(8):1706–14.
43. Institute of Medicine. Beyond myalgic encephalomyelitis/chronic fatigue syndrome: redefining an illness. The National Academies Press; 2015. https://doi. org/10.17226/19012.
44. Dumont R, Richard V, Lorthe E, et al. A population-based serological study of post-COVID syndrome prevalence and risk factors in children and adolescents. Nat Commun 2022;13(1):7086.
45. Bowe B, Xie Y, Al-Aly Z. Acute and post-acute sequelae associated with SARS-CoV-2 reinfection. Nat Med 2022;28(11):2398–405.
46. Byambasuren O, Stehlik P, Clark J, et al. Effect of covid-19 vaccination on long covid: systematic review. BMJ Med 2023;2(1):e000385.
47. Xie Y, Choi T, Al-Aly Z. Association of Treatment With Nirmatrelvir and the Risk of Post–COVID-19 Condition. JAMA Intern Med 2023;183(6):554–64.
48. Verduzco-Gutierrez M, Estores IM, Graf MJP, et al. Models of Care for Post-acute COVID-19 Clinics. Am J Phys Med Rehabil 2021;100(12):1133–9.
49. Barshikar S, Laguerre M, Gordon P, et al. Integrated Care Models for Long Coronavirus Disease. Phys Med Rehabil Clin 2023. https://doi.org/10.1016/j.pmr.2023. 03.007.
50. Morrow AK, Ng R, Vargas G, et al. Post-acute/Long COVID in Pediatrics: Development of a Multidisciplinary Rehabilitation Clinic and Preliminary Case Series. Am J Phys Med Rehabil 2021;100(12):1140–7.
51. Herrera JE, Niehaus WN, Whiteson J, et al. Multidisciplinary collaborative consensus guidance statement on the assessment and treatment of fatigue in post-acute sequelae of SARS-CoV-2 infection (PASC) patients. Pm R 2021; 13(9):1027–43.
52. Blitshteyn S, Whiteson JH, Abramoff B, et al. Multi-disciplinary collaborative consensus guidance statement on the assessment and treatment of autonomic dysfunction in patients with post-acute sequelae of SARS-CoV-2 infection (PASC). PM&R 2022;14(10):1270–91.

53. Rowe K. Chronic Fatigue Syndrome/Myalgic Encephalomyelitis (CFS/ME) in Adolescents: Practical Guidance and Management Challenges. Adolesc Health Med Ther 2023;14:13–26.

54. Hyatt KH, Jacobson LB, Schneider VS. Comparison of 70 degrees tilt, LBNP, and passive standing as measrues of orthostatic tolerance. Aviat Space Environ Med 1975;46(6):801–8.

55. Roma M, Marden CL, Rowe PC. Passive standing tests for the office diagnosis of postural tachycardia syndrome: New methodological considerations. Fatigue Biomed Health Behav 2018;6(4):179–92.

56. Tana C, Bentivegna E, Cho SJ, et al. Long COVID headache. J Headache Pain 2022;23(1):93.

57. Moskatel LS, Smirnoff L. Protracted headache after COVID-19: A case series of 31 patients from a tertiary headache center. Headache 2022;62(7):903–7.

58. Rodrigues AN, Dias ARN, Paranhos ACM, et al. Headache in long COVID as disabling condition: A clinical approach. Front Neurol 2023;14. Available at: https://www.frontiersin.org/articles/10.3389/fneur.2023.1149294. [Accessed 15 September 2023].

59. Ravindran MK, Zheng Y, Timbol C, et al. Migraine headaches in Chronic Fatigue Syndrome (CFS): Comparison of two prospective cross-sectional studies. BMC Neurol 2011;11(1):30.

60. van Campen C, Linda MC, Visser FC. Orthostatic Intolerance in Long-Haul COVID after SARS-CoV-2: A Case-Control Comparison with Post-EBV and Insidious-Onset Myalgic Encephalomyelitis/Chronic Fatigue Syndrome Patients. Healthcare 2022;10(10):2058.

61. Stewart JM, Gewitz MH, Weldon A, et al. Orthostatic Intolerance in Adolescent Chronic Fatigue Syndrome. Pediatrics 1999;103(1):116–21.

62. Bou-Holaigah I, Rowe PC, Kan J, et al. The relationship between neurally mediated hypotension and the chronic fatigue syndrome. JAMA 1995;274(12):961–7.

63. Afrin LB, Weinstock LB, Molderings GJ. Covid-19 hyperinflammation and post-Covid-19 illness may be rooted in mast cell activation syndrome. Int J Infect Dis 2020;100:327–32.

64. Gavrilova N, Soprun L, Lukashenko M, et al. New clinical phenotype of the post-covid syndrome: fibromyalgia and joint hypermobility condition. Pathophysiology 2022;29(1):24–9.

65. Barron DF, Cohen BA, Geraghty MT, et al. Joint hypermobility is more common in children with chronic fatigue syndrome than in healthy controls. J Pediatr 2002; 141(3):421–5.

66. Rowe PC, Barron DF, Calkins H, et al. Orthostatic intolerance and chronic fatigue syndrome associated with Ehlers-Danlos syndrome. J Pediatr 1999;135(4): 494–9.

67. Rowe PC, Marden CL, Heinlein S, et al. Improvement of severe myalgic encephalomyelitis/chronic fatigue syndrome symptoms following surgical treatment of cervical spinal stenosis. J Transl Med 2018;16(1):21.

68. Henderson FC, Rosenbaum R, Narayanan M, et al. Atlanto-axial rotary instability (Fielding type 1): characteristic clinical and radiological findings, and treatment outcomes following alignment, fusion, and stabilization. Neurosurg Rev 2021; 44(3):1553–68.

69. Rowe PC, Marden CL, Flaherty MAK, et al. Impaired range of motion of limbs and spine in chronic fatigue syndrome. J Pediatr 2014;165(2):360–6.

70. Knuttinen MG, Zurcher KS, Khurana N, et al. Imaging findings of pelvic venous insufficiency in patients with postural orthostatic tachycardia syndrome. Phlebology 2021;36(1):32–7.

71. Sandmann W, Scholbach T, Verginis K. Surgical treatment of abdominal compression syndromes: The significance of hypermobility-related disorders. Am J Med Genet C Semin Med Genet 2021;187(4):570–8.

72. Petracek LS, Broussard CA, Swope RL, et al. A Case Study of Successful Application of the Principles of ME/CFS Care to an Individual with Long COVID. Healthcare 2023;11(6):865.

73. Garg A, Subramain M, Barlow PB, et al. Patient Experiences with a Tertiary Care Post-COVID-19 Clinic. J Patient Exp 2023;10. https://doi.org/10.1177/237437 35231151539.

74. Bailey J, Lavelle B, Miller J, et al. Multidisciplinary Center Care for Long COVID Syndrome – a Retrospective Cohort Study. Am J Med 2023. https://doi.org/10.1016/j.amjmed.2023.05.002.

75. Varni JW, Seid M, Kurtin PS. PedsQL 4.0: reliability and validity of the Pediatric Quality of Life Inventory version 4.0 generic core scales in healthy and patient populations. Med Care 2001;39(8):800–12.

76. Varni JW, Limbers CA. The PedsQL Multidimensional Fatigue Scale in young adults: feasibility, reliability and validity in a University student population. Qual Life Res Int J Qual Life Asp Treat Care Rehabil 2008;17(1):105–14.

77. Rabin R, de Charro F. EQ-5D: a measure of health status from the EuroQol Group. Ann Med 2001;33(5):337–43.

78. Ghali A, Lacombe V, Ravaiau C, et al. The relevance of pacing strategies in managing symptoms of post-COVID-19 syndrome. J Transl Med 2023;21:375.

79. Casson S, Jones MD, Cassar J, et al. The effectiveness of activity pacing interventions for people with chronic fatigue syndrome: a systematic review and meta-analysis. Disabil Rehabil 2022;0(0):1–15.

80. Rowe K. Paediatric patients with myalgic encephalomyelitis/chronic fatigue syndrome value understanding and help to move on with their lives. Acta Paediatr 2020;109(4):790–800.

81. Bonilla H, Quach TC, Tiwari A, et al. Myalgic Encephalomyelitis/Chronic Fatigue Syndrome is common in post-acute sequelae of SARS-CoV-2 infection (PASC): Results from a post-COVID-19 multidisciplinary clinic. Front Neurol 2023;14. Available at: https://www.frontiersin.org/articles/10.3389/fneur.2023.1090747. [Accessed 14 September 2023].

82. Root T. Long Covid is said to affect white middle-aged women more – but data suggests otherwise. Guardian 2022. Available at: https://www.theguardian.com/society/2022/oct/14/long-covid-care-access. [Accessed 14 September 2023].

83. Lamas DJ. Opinion | Where Are All Our Post-Covid Patients? N Y Times 2022. Available at: https://www.nytimes.com/2022/09/26/opinion/post-covid-care.html. [Accessed 14 September 2023].

84. Eligulashvili A, Darrell M, Miller C, et al. COVID-19 Patients in the COVID-19 Recovery and Engagement (CORE) Clinics in the Bronx. Diagn Basel Switz 2022; 13(1):119.

85. Chatwani B, Flaherty S, Liu S, et al. 289. Post COVID Syndrome Cohort Characterization. Open Forum Infect Dis 2021;8(Suppl 1):S251–2.

86. Xie Y, Bowe B, Al-Aly Z. Burdens of post-acute sequelae of COVID-19 by severity of acute infection, demographics and health status. Nat Commun 2021;12(1): 6571.

87. RECOVER Initative. A Multi-Center Observational Study: The RECOVER Post Acute Sequelae of SARS-CoV-2 (PASC) Pediatric Cohort Study. 2022. Available at: https://www.niehs.nih.gov/research/programs/disaster/database/24282_main_508.pdf. [Accessed 14 September 2023].
88. Wyatt R, Laderman M, Botwinick L, et al. Achieving Health Equity: A Guide for Health Care Organizations. 2016. Available at: https://www.ihi.org/resources/Pages/IHIWhitePapers/Achieving-Health-Equity.aspx. [Accessed 14 September 2023].
89. The Future Pediatric Subspecialty Physician Workforce. Meeting the needs of infants, children, and adolescents. National Academies Press; 2023. https://doi.org/10.17226/27207.
90. Landon BE, Onnela JP, Meneades L, et al. Assessment of racial disparities in primary care physician specialty referrals. JAMA Netw Open 2021;4(1):e2029238.

Disordered Eating/Eating Disorders in Adolescents

Sydney M. Hartman-Munick, MD[a,*], Suzanne Allen, MSN, CPNP[b],
Anne Powell, MD[a]

KEYWORDS

- Eating disorder • Adolescent • Telehealth • Pandemic

KEY POINTS

- The volume and severity of eating disorders (EDs) increased among adolescents associated with the pandemic.
- There were several likely contributors to the rise in EDs among adolescents, including new pandemic-related stressors and absence of supports.
- Telehealth treatment was prevalent in the pandemic and patients, families, and providers had mixed feelings about the switch to virtual care.

INTRODUCTION
Definitions

Eating disorders (EDs), which are often diagnosed during adolescence, can profoundly impact adolescent development from both a physical and psychological standpoint.[1–3] EDs, which include anorexia nervosa, bulimia nervosa, other specified feeding/eating disorder, avoidant restrictive food intake disorder, and binge eating disorder, are associated with medical complications and are linked with elevated mortality rates when compared with the general population.[4,5] Up to 10% of individuals may struggle with an ED during their lifetime, and evidence suggests that rates of EDs have been increasing over time even prior to the onset of the coronavirus disease 2019 (COVID-19) pandemic.[2,6,7] Also of concern are disordered eating behaviors (DEBs), which can include caloric restriction, purging by vomiting, laxative misuse, excessive exercise, diet pill or muscle-building supplement use, and binge eating. These behaviors alone may not rise to the level of an ED diagnosis but can be dangerous and may predict the development of an ED later in life.[8] Recent research demonstrates that up to 20% of youth globally may engage in DEBs.[9]

[a] University of Massachusetts Memorial Children's Medical Center, UMass Chan Medical School, 55 Lake Avenue North, Worcester, MA 01655, USA; [b] University of Massachusetts Memorial Children's Medical Center, UMass Chan Medical School, Tan Chingfen Graduate School of Nursing, 55 Lake Avenue North, Worcester, MA 01655, USA
* Corresponding author.
E-mail address: sydney.hartman-munick@umassmemorial.org

Pediatr Clin N Am 71 (2024) 631–643
https://doi.org/10.1016/j.pcl.2024.04.005
0031-3955/24/© 2024 Elsevier Inc. All rights reserved.
pediatric.theclinics.com

Background

Medical complications of EDs are varied and numerous; the most common include bradycardia, electrolyte abnormalities, amenorrhea in those with a uterus, orthostatic vital sign changes, and syncope.[4] Psychiatric comorbidities are common among those with EDs, including depression, anxiety, obsessive compulsive disorder, substance use disorder, post-traumatic stress disorder, and personality disorders.[2,10–12] Those with EDs are at higher risk for suicide than their peers; this is particularly true for those with anorexia nervosa.[13,14]

Treatment for EDs generally involves a multidisciplinary approach with involvement of a medical provider, dietitian, and therapist.[15] The goals of ED treatment involve weight restoration if weight loss was a primary component of the ED pathology, as well as normalization of eating patterns and improvement in ED-related cognitions and behaviors.[15] While most patients are appropriate for outpatient specialist care, some patients benefit from higher levels of ED care via programs including intensive outpatient (evening), partial hospitalization (day), or residential programming.[4] When medical complications are present or malnutrition is severe, hospitalization for medical stabilization may be necessary and standard of care entails supervised feeding with an interdisciplinary approach involving medical, nutrition, psychology, and psychiatry providers.[4,15]

Individuals of any race, ethnicity, body size, socioeconomic status, gender identity, and sexual orientation may be at risk to develop an ED; however, those who do not fit the stereotype of the thin white female are less likely to receive adequate diagnosis and treatment, and may be more likely to have negative treatment experiences.[16–23] While prompt recognition of ED signs and symptoms is important for timely treatment, patients frequently face several structural barriers to appropriate care, which can be due to insurance coverage limitations/cost, geographic scarcity, and language or cultural barriers among others.[16,24,25]

DISCUSSION

Shortly after the onset of the COVID-19 pandemic, which quickly overwhelmed health care systems, providers began to anecdotally note increases in requests for evaluations, emergency room visits, and inpatient admissions for patients with EDs. These observations motivated a plethora of research on the trends in volume and characteristics of patients seeking care for EDs pre-onset and post-onset of the pandemic. The data demonstrate that the COVID-19 pandemic was associated with the development and worsening of ED symptoms in adolescents, both within North America and globally.[26]

Increases in Eating Disorders Among Adolescents in the Setting of the Pandemic

Hospitals throughout the United States and Canada[27] saw significant increases in medical hospitalizations for patients with EDs after onset of the pandemic.[28–31] One study that examined 14 hospital-based, geographically diverse adolescent medicine programs found that admissions more than doubled across all sites after onset of the pandemic.[32] With respect to outpatient evaluations that same study noted significant increases over time in outpatient assessments for EDs after onset of the pandemic.[32] While data through 2021 showed that both inpatient admissions and outpatient evaluations started to decline after the initial spike, these numbers are still well above pre-pandemic baselines.[32] The pandemic also correlated with significant increases in volume of emergency room visits for EDs; this trend mirrored that of inpatient and outpatient ED volume as well with an initial spike and subsequent decline in

2021 with numbers remaining well above their pre-pandemic baseline.[33] Data published by the Centers for Disease Control and Prevention noted that from 2019 to 2022, there was a doubling in the number of Emergency Department visits for patients' aged 12 to 17 with EDs.[34] A recent study demonstrated that patients with anorexia nervosa represented the highest percentage of patients admitted to the hospital for their ED, though this study also noted considerable increases in hospitalizations for patients with avoidant restrictive food intake disorder as well.[35]

Adolescent Patients with Eating Disorders Were Disproportionally Impacted by Coronavirus Disease 2019 Compared with Adults

While adult populations also saw increases in ED volume during the pandemic, evidence suggests that adolescent ED volume increases were significantly higher; a review noted an average increase of 83% in pediatric ED admissions, compared with an increase of 16% for adult admissions after onset of the pandemic.[26] A Canadian analysis of ED-related hospitalizations in children 10 to 19 years old revealed age differences even among adolescents, with higher numbers of teens aged 10 to 14 admitted with EDs in the first year of the pandemic and higher numbers of teens aged 15 to 19 with EDs admitted during the second.[36]

Severity of Illness and Length of Stay

In addition to the surge in volume of youth requiring care for EDs, patients with EDs tended to present with more severe illness and require longer hospitalizations during the pandemic.[31,37] Patients who reported the pandemic as a specific trigger for their ED were more likely to be medically unstable at presentation compared with patients who cited a non-pandemic-related onset.[37] Compared with pre-pandemic, patients who presented during the pandemic were also found to have lower average percentage of target goal weight at presentation and were 31% more likely to require hospital admission within 4 weeks of initial assessment.[37] In youth requiring hospitalization, ED symptoms at the time of admission, such as level of restriction and overexercising, were significantly higher in groups with EDs that started post-onset of the pandemic.[37,38] Rates of co-morbid psychiatric conditions, such as anxiety and depression, were also significantly higher in these patients.[28,38]

Length of hospital stay for adolescent patients with EDs also increased post-onset of the pandemic. Examination across 38 hospitals revealed that the total cumulative bed days for patients with EDs was 40,933 in the 27 months pre-pandemic, compared with 67,907 bed days in the 27 months post-onset of the pandemic.[33] Data also suggest that patients hospitalized after onset of the pandemic were more likely to require rapid readmission after discharge, with a study indicating such patients were 8.68 times more likely to be readmitted within 30 days of discharge compared with those first hospitalized pre-pandemic.[29]

Global Trends in Eating Disorders in the Setting of the Pandemic

Increases in adolescents with EDs were observed on a global scale. A 2023 systematic review examined 53 studies from around the world that looked at changes in volume of ED patients in association with the pandemic.[26] A pooled average across 11 studies showed a 48% increase in the number of hospital admissions during the pandemic compared to a similar time frame the preceding year.[26] In a study examining the patterns of admission rates and symptom severity of childhood and adolescent anorexia nervosa in Europe, hospitals in Spain, France, Italy, and the Netherlands showed an increase in ED-related admissions.[39] In addition, clinicians at these programs estimated that patients' symptom severity was increased compared with prior to the onset of the pandemic.[39]

Reasons for Increases in Eating Disorders Among Adolescents During the Pandemic

It has been well established that stressful life events may contribute to the development of EDs among youth. This can include major changes in school, family, relationships, home, health, and/or safety.[40] Combined with other risk factors for EDs such as genetic predisposition, body dissatisfaction, low self-esteem, history of trauma, individual coping skills, societal and familial expectations, body image ideals, and structural inequities such as homophobia, transphobia, and racism, the pandemic and its associated changes likely put adolescents in a vulnerable position with respect to the development of EDs.[41–46] Research indicates that pandemic-associated increases in EDs among adolescents were secondary to a wide range of factors, both on a broad and individual scale (**Fig. 1**). This includes both exposure to increased risk factors for EDs, as well as decreased access to protective factors that may reduce the risk of EDs.[47]

Pandemic-Associated Risk Factors for Eating Disorders

The widespread impacts of the pandemic and the mitigation strategies implemented to prevent the spread of the virus led to many rapid societal changes that may have increased risk for the development of EDs. The sudden onset of the pandemic and risk of significant illness and death led to anxiety, uncertainty, and grief around the world, all of which are known to be associated with the development of EDs.[47,48] One study noted an association between higher levels of COVID-19-related anxiety and uncertainty with increased ED severity among college students.[49] Similarly, difficulties with stress management and increased depression were found to be associated with unhealthy weight control behaviors among young adults during the pandemic.[50]

Simultaneous with the increases in stress, uncertainty, and anxiety, efforts to stop the spread of COVID-19 led to mandated social isolation.[51] The impact on adolescents and young adults was immediate with school closures and a switch to remote schooling leading to significantly decreased social interactions.[52] This isolation, combined with an increase in stress, anxiety, and grief developed into a perfect storm for the exacerbation or development of EDs.[47,48] One qualitative study of social media posts during the pandemic noted themes of isolation as a trigger for compulsive exercise, a concern that was echoed in an additional study of patients with anorexia

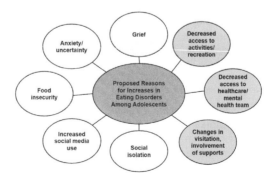

Fig. 1. Proposed reasons for increases in eating disorder (ED) volume among adolescents during the coronavirus disease 2019 (COVID-19) pandemic[a]. [a]Yellow corresponds with presence of risk factors for EDs, green corresponds with absence of protective factors.

nervosa.[53,54] Another study cited the feeling of being "imprisoned" as it connected to lower motivation to work on recovery.[55]

Mandated social isolation forced people around the world to turn to virtual interactions including remote school and work which dramatically changed routines and social interactions. During this time, the use of social media among adolescents increased.[53,56] Early into the pandemic, both mainstream and social media coverage included a new anxiety: the "Quarantine 15," which referenced a fear of weight gain in the setting of social isolation using messaging riddled with anti-fat bias.[48,50,53,55] Though some online interactions were found to be positive for creating supportive communities around ED recovery, there was also evidence that exposure to negative ED-specific social media increased among adolescent populations.[53,56,57] In addition to increased social media use, prolonged periods of time on virtual platforms for school with students staring at their own images on camera likely contributed to body image concerns.[57]

Additionally, the pandemic led to lost jobs, supply chain interruptions, and economic instability which had negative impacts on the availability of food.[58] Food insecurity is a known risk factor for the development of and exacerbation of disordered eating behaviors, even among those without a prior ED history.[48] Uncertainty regarding the availability of food and decreased access to safe foods triggered ED pathology including restricting, delaying eating, eating less, bingeing, and purging.[50] Changes in food availability also led to increased ED pathology such as obsessive cleaning and fear of food through the fear of contamination.[55]

Pandemic Impacts on Protective Factors

While increased social isolation likely contributed to the development of EDs among adolescents, lack of access to protective factors such as clubs, sports, hobbies, healthy exercise, travel, and supportive adults may be implicated as well.[50,55] In addition, decreased access to health care providers led to strains on those in treatment for EDs as well as for healthy adolescents.[48,53,55,59] Rapidly changing guidelines and stay-at-home orders saw a decrease in health care utilization among patients with EDs.[54] One study found that in-person outpatient psychotherapy decreased from 88.1% to 55.3%, being weighed by a clinician decreased from 48.4% to 30.8%, and 10.7% of patients stopped therapy completely during the pandemic.[54] Patients and families also reported difficulties with outpatient and inpatient ED treatment because of less contact with their treatment team, lack of available ED providers, ED programs at capacity, insurance barriers, and decreased income.[55,59] Strict visitation rules also increased stress for those participating in residential care, as often only 1 family member was allowed to visit, putting pressure on that individual and decreasing the patient's access to multiple supports outside of treatment.[55,59]

While studies show a link between the onset of the pandemic and decreased protective factors against EDs among adolescents, many teens called upon unique strategies to cope and protect themselves from new or worsening ED symptoms during that time. One study that examined coping strategies for mental health among teens in the pandemic noted that the most common strategies used were maintenance of social ties, relaxation, use of routine, and keeping busy.[60] Participants in a qualitative study discussed being particular about filtering social media such that they were seeing more positive content, or avoiding social media altogether.[57] Others noted that coming together with loved ones and creating their own structure and routine to stay busy, as well as maintaining their meal plans was helpful in combatting worsening ED symptoms.[57]

CHALLENGES/OPPORTUNITIES RELATING TO TELEHEALTH
The Shift to Virtual Care

Early in the pandemic, most states in the United States rolled out stay-at-home orders, and several Canadian provinces had varying levels of COVID-related restrictions as well.[61] While recommendations varied between institutions, most hospitals and outpatient medical centers had some limitations on both visits and types of hospital admissions, such as non-urgent visits or elective procedures, respectively.[62,63] The immediate decline in outpatient visits left a gap in ED care for many patients, and ED providers of all types had to rapidly shift to providing telehealth appointments. With this shift, came barriers to overcome including telehealth platform training for providers, development of new protocols for triage, facilitating patient access to the telehealth platform, and availability of technological support for issues during remote visits.[64] While many sites were able to quickly implement the use of virtual visits, there was still a lag time and many patients with EDs had disruption in their access to care to some degree.[65,66] Non-hospital-based ED programs had similar shifts to telehealth, with some programs changing to fully virtual intensive outpatient and partial hospitalization programming. In the inpatient hospital setting, some psychiatry services shifted to doing virtual sessions with patients admitted for ED treatment as well.[67] This rapid scale up was an adjustment for providers, patients, and families and experiences were varied.

The Patient/Family Perspective

While studies have shown that the use of telehealth is generally acceptable to teens,[68,69] experiences were mixed regarding the shift to virtual ED care (**Fig. 2**). Teen patients overall did well with adapting to a telehealth platform logistically, though 1 con cited was the difficulty when technology glitched and visits cut out right in the middle of a vulnerable moment.[70] Experiences were deemed distinctly worse for those who had trouble accessing the technology, and research has shown that this burden has tended to fall on individuals who already face barriers to treatment including

	Pros	Cons
Patient/Family	Continued meal support, psychoeducation	Technological glitches
	Decreased cost	Difficult to be emotionally vulnerable virtually
	Reduced travel burden	Easier to hide setbacks/avoid difficult conversations
	Ease of use for adolescents	Less able to achieve therapeutic breakthroughs
	Availability of team	Privacy/confidentiality concerns
Provider	Increased family involvement	Easier for patients to disengage emotionally
	Ability to meet frequently as a team	More difficult to monitor medical stability
	More time for patient to enjoy life outside of ED treatment	Privacy/ confidentiality concerns
	Increased individualization of treatment	Technological glitches
	No room or space limitations	Professional isolation/lack of camaraderie
	Increased availability of professional supervision	Harder to monitor patient behaviors/emotions throughout the day
	Easier access to professional didactic sessions	Logistically more difficult to provide meal support

Fig. 2. Pros and cons of virtual treatment for adolescents with EDs during the COVID-19 pandemic: Patient/family and provider perspectives.

racially minortized individuals and those of lower socioeconomic status.[70–72] Others described that it was more difficult to open up over telehealth than in person, and potentially easier to hide setbacks or struggles.[66,73,74] Despite this, most patients and families rated virtual programming as helpful, often praising availability of the team and the flexibility of virtual care as positives.[70,73,74] Other bonuses to telehealth programming included decreased cost of care in part due to reduced travel burden.[74] Families noted that virtual care seemed to be helpful for the practical aspects of recovery, such as meal advice or psychoeducation for parents, but less so for the deeper work of therapeutic breakthroughs.[70]

Though many patients cited virtual care as helpful, in a study, two-thirds of patients stated they would not choose to continue with virtual treatment, and half noted they would not recommend it to family or friends.[75] Further, patients who had started therapy in person and then switched to virtual with the onset of the pandemic felt that therapeutically the virtual treatment was inferior.[70,75] Lastly, concerns have been raised regarding telehealth and privacy/confidentiality, neither of which can be absolutely assured in the telehealth setting given the provider's lack of control over the environment and the fact that family members were often home during the pandemic alongside their children.[64] Overall, while perceptions of virtual ED care were clearly varied, there was a frequent theme among studies that virtual care for EDs was better than not having care at all.[70,73]

The Provider Perspective

Like the patient and family experience, perspectives on the switch to virtual care from ED providers were mixed (see **Fig. 2**). One study that surveyed staff in an ED partial hospitalization program revealed concerns that it was much easier to disengage when on a screen, so this modality might not be the best for patients with lower motivation or who were struggling.[76] That study also cited concerns that monitoring physical health and for medical decompensation was much more difficult, which was echoed by another study examining provider perspective.[74,76] Confidentiality concerns as well as issues with technology glitches were raised as well, and some reported worries about the professional isolation of virtual treatment, which does not provide an opportunity to walk down the hall and run a case by a colleague for their thoughts.[74,76] Some providers noted logistical concerns, such as the inability to really provide concrete meal support when not sitting next to a patient, or worries about not having eyes on the patient in between sessions like they would when the patient was there all day in person (though interestingly, another provider stated they felt it was helpful for patients to have less hours engaging in their program and more time to enjoy life outside of their ED).[76] Despite these challenges, providers cited positives to virtual ED care, including the ability for the family to be more involved by reducing transportation barriers, and for the entire team to meet regularly.[76] Some providers noted that the virtual model allowed them to be more flexible with their support and to individualize treatment better, such as providing support after meals, using different varieties of group therapy, and not being limited by room availability or space.[74,76] From a professional development standpoint, another study cited the expanded ability for provider supervision for learning via virtual platforms, as well as increased access to didactics for learning as positives to the virtual environment.[67]

Patient Outcomes

Several studies examined short-term (less than or equal to 1 year) outcomes comparing telehealth with in-person ED treatment, and results are promising with respect to the potential efficacy of virtual ED treatment, though sample sizes for most of these studies have been small. Studies consistently demonstrated significant increases in body mass index (BMI), and improvement in ED symptoms and mood symptoms with the use of virtual ED treatment modalities.[66,77–79] Two studies compared outcomes from virtual treatment with in-person treatment by incorporating pre-pandemic data and found that there were no significant differences in BMI increases, ED symptoms, depression and perfectionism scores, or need for hospitalization 6 months after the end of the program.[77,78] One study noted a longer duration of treatment with virtual ED care; however, at the same time, reported that the treatment intensity was lower as was the cost of treatment based on billing.[78] Longer term studies are needed with larger sample sizes to further compare in person versus virtual ED care; however, these initial results are encouraging for potentially expanding access to care for many patients and families.

SUMMARY

Adolescents faced pervasive and unique stressors in the setting of the COVID-19 pandemic.[47–50] These stressors were associated with a significant rise in the number of adolescents with EDs around the world and may have contributed to increased severity of presentation and longer hospital stays seen in the pandemic as well.[28–34,37] Treatment teams adapted quickly to virtual care, and while this is a promising model for delivery of ED treatment, it may not be effective for all patients, and an increase in the workforce of specialists with ED expertise will be necessary to meet the demands of this vulnerable population.[70–76] Given the acuity of these patients as well as the natural history of EDs, the health care system is likely to feel the effects of this pandemic-related rise in patient volume and severity for years to come.

CLINICS CARE POINTS

- Pandemic-related stressors such as isolation, stress/anxiety, and food insecurity contributed to the development/worsening of EDs among adolescents
- Strategies to help combat these crisis-related stressors and foster resilience include maintenance of social ties, routine and structure, and avoidance or strategic use of social media
- Adolescents saw significant increases in volume and severity of patients with EDs in the setting of the pandemic
- Telehealth is a promising treatment intervention for EDs but has not been universally accepted
- In the event of another large-scale crisis that results in limitations on in-person visits, practices should have in place methods to quickly scale up virtual interactions with regular check-ins with patients, particularly those at risk for mental health concerns

DISCLOSURE

The authors have nothing to disclose.

REFERENCES

1. Tanner AB. Unique considerations for the medical care of restrictive eating disorders in children and young adolescents. J Eat Disord 2023;11(1):33.

2. Herpertz-Dahlmann B. Adolescent eating disorders: update on definitions, symptomatology, epidemiology, and comorbidity. Child Adolesc Psychiatr Clin N Am 2015;24(1):177–96.
3. Solmi M, Radua J, Olivola M, et al. Age at onset of mental disorders worldwide: large-scale meta-analysis of 192 epidemiological studies. Mol Psychiatr 2022; 27(1):281–95.
4. Hornberger LL, Lane MA, COMMITTEE ON ADOLESCENCE. Identification and Management of Eating Disorders in Children and Adolescents. Pediatrics 2021; 147(1):e2020040279. https://doi.org/10.1542/peds.2020-040279.
5. Arcelus J, Mitchell AJ, Wales J, et al. Mortality rates in patients with anorexia nervosa and other eating disorders. A meta-analysis of 36 studies. Arch Gen Psychiatr 2011;68(7):724–31.
6. Galmiche M, Déchelotte P, Lambert G, et al. Prevalence of eating disorders over the 2000-2018 period: a systematic literature review. Am J Clin Nutr 2019;109(5): 1402–13.
7. van Eeden AE, van Hoeken D, Hoek HW. Incidence, prevalence and mortality of anorexia nervosa and bulimia nervosa. Curr Opin Psychiatr 2021;34(6):515–24.
8. Neumark-Sztainer D, Wall M, Guo J, et al. Obesity, disordered eating, and eating disorders in a longitudinal study of adolescents: how do dieters fare 5 years later? J Am Diet Assoc 2006;106(4):559–68.
9. López-Gil JF, García-Hermoso A, Smith L, et al. Global Proportion of Disordered Eating in Children and Adolescents: A Systematic Review and Meta-analysis. JAMA Pediatr 2023;177(4):363–72.
10. Bahji A, Mazhar MN, Hudson CC, et al. Prevalence of substance use disorder comorbidity among individuals with eating disorders: A systematic review and meta-analysis. Psychiatr Res 2019;273:58–66.
11. Shah R, Zanarini MC. Comorbidity of Borderline Personality Disorder: Current Status and Future Directions. Psychiatr Clin 2018;41(4):583–93.
12. Rijkers C, Schoorl M, van Hoeken D, et al. Eating disorders and posttraumatic stress disorder. Curr Opin Psychiatr 2019;32(6):510–7.
13. Smith AR, Zuromski KL, Dodd DR. Eating disorders and suicidality: what we know, what we don't know, and suggestions for future research. Curr Opin Psychol 2018;22:63–7.
14. Cliffe C, Shetty H, Himmerich H, et al. Suicide attempts requiring hospitalization in patients with eating disorders: A retrospective cohort study. Int J Eat Disord 2020; 53(5):458–65.
15. Society for Adolescent Health and Medicine, Golden NH, Katzman DK, et al. Position Paper of the Society for Adolescent Health and Medicine: medical management of restrictive eating disorders in adolescents and young adults. J Adolesc Health 2015;56(1):121–5.
16. Moreno R, Buckelew SM, Accurso EC, et al. Disparities in access to eating disorders treatment for publicly-insured youth and youth of color: a retrospective cohort study. J Eat Disord 2023;11(1):10.
17. Sonneville KR, Lipson SK. Disparities in eating disorder diagnosis and treatment according to weight status, race/ethnicity, socioeconomic background, and sex among college students. Int J Eat Disord 2018;51(6):518–26.
18. Mikhail ME, Klump KL. A virtual issue highlighting eating disorders in people of black/African and Indigenous heritage. Int J Eat Disord 2021;54(3):459–67.
19. Cheng ZH, Perko VL, Fuller-Marashi L, et al. Ethnic differences in eating disorder prevalence, risk factors, and predictive effects of risk factors among young women. Eat Behav 2019;32:23–30.

20. Vo M, Golden N. Medical complications and management of atypical anorexia nervosa. J Eat Disord 2022;10(1):196.

21. Diemer EW, Grant JD, Munn-Chernoff MA, et al. Gender Identity, Sexual Orientation, and Eating-Related Pathology in a National Sample of College Students. J Adolesc Health 2015;57(2):144–9.

22. Calzo JP, Blashill AJ, Brown TA, et al. Eating Disorders and Disordered Weight and Shape Control Behaviors in Sexual Minority Populations. Curr Psychiatr Rep 2017;19(8):49.

23. Hernández JC, Perez M, Hoek HW. Update on the epidemiology and treatment of eating disorders among Hispanic/Latinx Americans in the United States. Curr Opin Psychiatr 2022;35(6):379–84.

24. Thompson C, Park S. Barriers to access and utilization of eating disorder treatment among women. Arch Womens Ment Health 2016;19(5):753–60.

25. Johns G, Taylor B, John A, et al. Current eating disorder healthcare services - the perspectives and experiences of individuals with eating disorders, their families and health professionals: systematic review and thematic synthesis. BJPsych Open 2019;5(4):e59.

26. J Devoe D, Han A, Anderson A, et al. The impact of the COVID-19 pandemic on eating disorders: A systematic review. Int J Eat Disord 2023;56(1):5–25.

27. Toigo S, Katzman DK, Vyver E, et al. Eating disorder hospitalizations among children and youth in Canada from 2010 to 2022: a population-based surveillance study using administrative data. J Eat Disord 2024;12(1):3.

28. Feldman MA, King CK, Vitale S, et al. The impact of COVID-19 on adolescents with eating disorders: Increased need for medical stabilization and decreased access to care. Int J Eat Disord 2023;56(1):257–62.

29. Matthews A, Kramer RA, Peterson CM, et al. Higher admission and rapid readmission rates among medically hospitalized youth with anorexia nervosa/atypical anorexia nervosa during COVID-19. Eat Behav 2021;43:101573. https://doi.org/10.1016/j.eatbeh.2021.101573.

30. Otto AK, Jary JM, Sturza J, et al. Medical Admissions Among Adolescents With Eating Disorders During the COVID-19 Pandemic [published correction appears in Pediatrics. 2022 Jan 1;149(1):]. Pediatrics 2021;148(4):e2021052201. https://doi.org/10.1542/peds.2021-052201.

31. Lin JA, Hartman-Munick SM, Kells MR, et al. The Impact of the COVID-19 Pandemic on the Number of Adolescents/Young Adults Seeking Eating Disorder-Related Care. J Adolesc Health 2021;69(4):660–3.

32. Hartman-Munick SM, Lin JA, Milliren CE, et al. Association of the COVID-19 Pandemic With Adolescent and Young Adult Eating Disorder Care Volume. JAMA Pediatr 2022;176(12):1225–32.

33. Milliren CE, Richmond TK, Hudgins JD. Emergency Department Visits and Hospitalizations for Eating Disorders During the COVID-19 Pandemic. Pediatrics 2023;151(1):e2022058198. https://doi.org/10.1542/peds.2022-058198.

34. Radhakrishnan L, Leeb RT, Bitsko RH, et al. Pediatric Emergency Department Visits Associated with Mental Health Conditions Before and During the COVID-19 Pandemic - United States, January 2019-January 2022. MMWR Morb Mortal Wkly Rep 2022;71(8):319–24.

35. Rappaport DI, O'Connor M, Reedy C, Vo M. Clinical Characteristics of US Adolescents Hospitalized for Eating Disorders 2010-2022. Hosp Pediatr 2024;14(1):52–8.

36. Auger N, Steiger H, Luu TM, et al. Shifting age of child eating disorder hospitalizations during the Covid-19 pandemic. J Child Psychol Psychiatry 2023;64(8): 1176–84.

37. Spettigue W, Obeid N, Erbach M, et al. The impact of COVID-19 on adolescents with eating disorders: a cohort study. J Eat Disord 2021;9(1):65.

38. Schreyer CC, Vanzhula IA, Guarda AS. Evaluating the impact of COVID-19 on severity at admission and response to inpatient treatment for adult and adolescent patients with eating disorders. Int J Eat Disord 2023;56(1):182–91.

39. Gilsbach S, Plana MT, Castro-Fornieles J, et al. Increase in admission rates and symptom severity of childhood and adolescent anorexia nervosa in Europe during the COVID-19 pandemic: data from specialized eating disorder units in different European countries. Child Adolesc Psychiatr Ment Health 2022;16(1):46.

40. Berge JM, Loth K, Hanson C, et al. Family life cycle transitions and the onset of eating disorders: a retrospective grounded theory approach. J Clin Nurs 2012; 21(9–10):1355–63.

41. Suarez-Albor CL, Galletta M, Gómez-Bustamante EM. Factors associated with eating disorders in adolescents: a systematic review. Acta Biomed 2022;93(3): e2022253. https://doi.org/10.23750/abm.v93i3.13140.

42. Culbert KM, Racine SE, Klump KL. Research Review: What we have learned about the causes of eating disorders - a synthesis of sociocultural, psychological, and biological research. J Child Psychol Psychiatry 2015;56(11):1141–64.

43. Uniacke B, Glasofer D, Devlin M, et al. Predictors of eating-related psychopathology in transgender and gender nonbinary individuals. Eat Behav 2021;42: 101527. https://doi.org/10.1016/j.eatbeh.2021.101527.

44. Convertino AD, Brady JP, Albright CA, et al. The role of sexual minority stress and community involvement on disordered eating, dysmorphic concerns and appearance- and performance-enhancing drug misuse. Body Image 2021;36:53–63.

45. Brown KL, Graham AK, Perera RA, et al. Eating to cope: Advancing our understanding of the effects of exposure to racial discrimination on maladaptive eating behaviors. Int J Eat Disord 2022;55(12):1744–52.

46. Convertino AD, Morland LA, Blashill AJ. Trauma exposure and eating disorders: Results from a United States nationally representative sample. Int J Eat Disord 2022;55(8):1079–89.

47. Rodgers RF, Lombardo C, Cerolini S, et al. The impact of the COVID-19 pandemic on eating disorder risk and symptoms. Int J Eat Disord 2020;53(7): 1166–70.

48. Cooper M, Reilly EE, Siegel JA, et al. Eating disorders during the COVID-19 pandemic and quarantine: an overview of risks and recommendations for treatment and early intervention. Eat Disord 2022;30(1):54–76.

49. Scharmer C, Martinez K, Gorrell S, et al. Eating disorder pathology and compulsive exercise during the COVID-19 public health emergency: Examining risk associated with COVID-19 anxiety and intolerance of uncertainty. Int J Eat Disord 2020;53(12):2049–54.

50. Simone M, Emery RL, Hazzard VM, et al. Disordered eating in a population-based sample of young adults during the COVID-19 outbreak. Int J Eat Disord 2021; 54(7):1189–201.

51. CDC museum COVID-19 timeline. Centers for Disease Control and Prevention; 2023. Available at: https://www.cdc.gov/museum/timeline/covid19.html. [Accessed 25 September 2023].

52. COVID experience surveys (CovEx). Centers for Disease Control and Prevention; 2023. Available at: https://www.cdc.gov/healthyyouth/data/covex/index.htm. [Accessed 25 September 2023].

53. Nutley SK, Falise AM, Henderson R, et al. Impact of the COVID-19 Pandemic on Disordered Eating Behavior: Qualitative Analysis of Social Media Posts. JMIR Ment Health 2021;8(1):e26011. https://doi.org/10.2196/26011.

54. Schlegl S, Maier J, Meule A, et al. Eating disorders in times of the COVID-19 pandemic-Results from an online survey of patients with anorexia nervosa. Int J Eat Disord 2020;53(11):1791–800.

55. Zeiler M, Wittek T, Kahlenberg L, et al. Impact of COVID-19 Confinement on Adolescent Patients with Anorexia Nervosa: A Qualitative Interview Study Involving Adolescents and Parents. Int J Environ Res Publ Health 2021;18(8): 4251.

56. Vall-Roqué H, Andrés A, Saldaña C. The impact of COVID-19 lockdown on social network sites use, body image disturbances and self-esteem among adolescent and young women. Prog Neuro-Psychopharmacol Biol Psychiatry 2021;110: 110293. https://doi.org/10.1016/j.pnpbp.2021.110293.

57. Fernández-Aranda F, Casas M, Claes L, et al. COVID-19 and implications for eating disorders. Eur Eat Disord Rev 2020 May;28(3):239–45.

58. Kim-Mozeleski JE, Pike Moore SN, Trapl ES, et al. Food Insecurity Trajectories in the US During the First Year of the COVID-19 Pandemic. Prev Chronic Dis 2023; 20:E03.

59. Goode RW, Godoy SM, Wolfe H, et al. Perceptions and experiences with eating disorder treatment in the first year of COVID-19: A longitudinal qualitative analysis. Int J Eat Disord 2023;56(1):247–56.

60. Waselewski EA, Waselewski ME, Chang T. Needs and Coping Behaviors of Youth in the U.S. During COVID-19. J Adolesc Health 2020;67(5):649–52.

61. Moreland A, Herlihy C, Tynan MA, et al. Timing of State and Territorial COVID-19 Stay-at-Home Orders and Changes in Population Movement - United States, March 1-May 31, 2020. MMWR Morb Mortal Wkly Rep 2020;69(35):1198–203.

62. Schweiberger K, Patel SY, Mehrotra A, et al. Trends in Pediatric Primary Care Visits During the Coronavirus Disease of 2019 Pandemic. Acad Pediatr 2021; 21(8):1426–33.

63. Pelletier JH, Rakkar J, Au AK, et al. Trends in US Pediatric Hospital Admissions in 2020 Compared With the Decade Before the COVID-19 Pandemic. JAMA Netw Open 2021;4(2):e2037227. https://doi.org/10.1001/jamanetworkopen.2020. 37227 [published correction appears in JAMA Netw Open. 2021 Apr 1;4(4): e2111979].

64. Barney A, Buckelew S, Mesheriakova V, et al. The COVID-19 Pandemic and Rapid Implementation of Adolescent and Young Adult Telemedicine: Challenges and Opportunities for Innovation. J Adolesc Health 2020;67(2):164–71.

65. Spigel R, Lin JA, Milliren CE, et al. Access to care and worsening eating disorder symptomatology in youth during the COVID-19 pandemic. J Eat Disord 2021; 9(1):69.

66. Plumley S, Kristensen A, Jenkins PE. Continuation of an eating disorders day programme during the COVID-19 pandemic. J Eat Disord 2021;9(1):34.

67. Datta N, Derenne J, Sanders M, et al. Telehealth transition in a comprehensive care unit for eating disorders: Challenges and long-term benefits. Int J Eat Disord 2020;53(11):1774–9.

68. Wood SM, Pickel J, Phillips AW, et al. Acceptability, Feasibility, and Quality of Telehealth for Adolescent Health Care Delivery During the COVID-19 Pandemic:

Cross-sectional Study of Patient and Family Experiences. JMIR Pediatr Parent 2021;4(4):e32708. https://doi.org/10.2196/32708.

69. Kodjebacheva GD, Culinski T, Kawser B, et al. Satisfaction with pediatric telehealth according to the opinions of children and adolescents during the COVID-19 pandemic: A literature review. Front Public Health 2023;11:1145486. https://doi.org/10.3389/fpubh.2023.1145486.

70. Stewart C, Konstantellou A, Kassamali F, et al. Is this the 'new normal'? A mixed method investigation of young person, parent and clinician experience of online eating disorder treatment during the COVID-19 pandemic. J Eat Disord 2021; 9(1):78.

71. Wood SM, White K, Peebles R, et al. Outcomes of a Rapid Adolescent Telehealth Scale-Up During the COVID-19 Pandemic. J Adolesc Health 2020;67(2):172–8.

72. Williams C, Shang D. Telehealth Usage Among Low-Income Racial and Ethnic Minority Populations During the COVID-19 Pandemic: Retrospective Observational Study. J Med Internet Res 2023;25:e43604. https://doi.org/10.2196/43604.

73. Brothwood PL, Baudinet J, Stewart CS, et al. Moving online: young people and parents' experiences of adolescent eating disorder day programme treatment during the COVID-19 pandemic. J Eat Disord 2021;9(1):62.

74. Shaw H, Robertson S, Ranceva N. What was the impact of a global pandemic (COVID-19) lockdown period on experiences within an eating disorder service? A service evaluation of the views of patients, parents/carers and staff. J Eat Disord 2021;9(1):14.

75. Lewis YD, Elran-Barak R, Grundman-Shem Tov R, et al. The abrupt transition from face-to-face to online treatment for eating disorders: a pilot examination of patients' perspectives during the COVID-19 lockdown. J Eat Disord 2021;9(1):31.

76. Webb H, Dalton B, Irish M, et al. Clinicians' perspectives on supporting individuals with severe anorexia nervosa in specialist eating disorder intensive treatment settings during the COVID-19 pandemic. J Eat Disord 2022;10(1):30.

77. Levinson CA, Spoor SP, Keshishian AC, et al. Pilot outcomes from a multidisciplinary telehealth versus in-person intensive outpatient program for eating disorders during versus before the Covid-19 pandemic. Int J Eat Disord 2021;54(9): 1672–9.

78. Van Huysse JL, Prohaska N, Miller C, et al. Adolescent eating disorder treatment outcomes of an in-person partial hospital program versus a virtual intensive outpatient program. Int J Eat Disord 2023;56(1):192–202.

79. Raykos BC, Erceg-Hurn DM, Hill J, et al. Positive outcomes from integrating telehealth into routine clinical practice for eating disorders during COVID-19. Int J Eat Disord 2021;54(9):1689–95.

Obesity

Post-Pandemic Weight Management

Annemarie McCartney Swamy, MD, PhD[a,b]

KEYWORDS

- Obesity • Weight loss • COVID-19 pandemic • Semaglutide • Bariatric surgery
- Weight stigma

KEY POINTS

- The coronavirus disease 2019 pandemic led to increased incidence of adolescents with obesity, mental health concerns, and disordered eating behaviors, as well as social media dialog around weight stigma and size bias.
- The American Academy of Pediatrics' new clinical practice guidelines recommend early inventions as opposed to "watchful waiting" when adolescents present with obesity.
- Intensive health behavior and lifestyle treatment is recommended for all patients, and some adolescents may also be offered anti-obesity medication and referred for bariatric surgery.
- Semaglutide was approved by the Food and Drug Administration for weight loss in adolescents in 2022 and is the most effective medication but is not covered by most insurance plans.

INTRODUCTION

Obesity in children and adolescents is defined as having a body mass index (BMI) greater than or equal to the 95th percentile relative to others of the same age and sex,[1] and it is associated with several comorbidities, including but not limited to cardiovascular disease, dyslipidemia, type 2 diabetes mellitus (T2DM), hyperinsulinism, asthma, sleep disorders, kidney disease, non-alcoholic steatohepatitis.[2,3] Further, there is an increased risk of complications from coronavirus disease 2019 (COVID-19) in those with obesity, and they are more likely to require respiratory support.[3] The pandemic highlighted and worsened socioeconomic disparities, especially in families who had previously been experiencing food insecurity, further increasing the risk of pediatric obesity in food-insecure settings.[2] Beyond physical effects of obesity, there is increased risk of depression, low self-esteem, disordered eating behavior, and lower educational achievement, in part due to weight stigma from peers, family, media, and

[a] Adolescent Medicine, Department of Pediatrics, Charleston Area Medical Center, 830 Pennsylvania Avenue, Suite 401, Charleston, WV 25302, USA; [b] West Virginia University
E-mail address: annemarie.swamy@hsc.wvu.edu

Pediatr Clin N Am 71 (2024) 645–652
https://doi.org/10.1016/j.pcl.2024.04.007   **pediatric.theclinics.com**
0031-3955/24/© 2024 Elsevier Inc. All rights reserved, including those for text and data mining, AI training, and similar technologies.

health care providers.[4] The effects of comorbidities of obesity in our young people can have a detrimental impact on the future workforce, as data suggest that adults with obesity can experience lost productivity.[5] Early treatment and prevention may reduce the prevalence of adults who have negative health effects related to excess weight, as more than half of prepubescent children with overweight become adults with overweight.[2]

Prior to the COVID-19 pandemic, approximately 19.3% of youths aged 2 to 19 years had obesity,[6] and clinics started to observe increases in children's and adolescents' weight and BMI as early as 3 months after the pandemic's onset.[7] Closures of school, gyms, and parks, combined with a transition to online learning and increased screen time, contributed to a more sedentary lifestyle.[8] Coupled with increased consumption of calorie-dense food, the prevalence of obesity increased,[9] with some clinics finding a 3.1% to 5.2% increase in 12-year-olds to 17 year-olds within the first year of the pandemic.[7] Although some families spent more time outdoors, disparities in access to safe, outdoor spaces for physical activity, especially in urban areas, may have contributed to increased weight gain in those with lower socioeconomic status.[8] Further, there was increased prevalence of food insecurity; with closures of schools, students lost access to free or reduced-price meals that had been provided at school.[10] Programs that were created to bridge the gap while maintaining social distancing may have contributed to over 50% of food-insecure families reporting an increase in processed food consumption.[10]

IMPACT OF SOCIAL MEDIA AND INTERNET USE

Social media use surged with the onset of the pandemic, perhaps in part due to reduced in-person social interactions imposed by the pandemic. Platforms such as TikTok and Instagram have become increasingly popular but are sources of dangerous "challenges" and weight-loss "hacks," and social media has contributed to weight stigma, particularly with the pervasive use of filters to create unrealistic, idealized photos and with anonymous weight-related attacks on individuals.[11] To a lesser degree, social media platforms have also been used to promote positive messaging such as highlighting diversity in body sizes and emphasizing body positivity.[11] Providers and parents should be aware of the types of media that youths consume, including whether they are seeking weight-related or size-related content, such as searching problematic hashtags like #weightloss, #whatleatinaday, #thinspiration/thinspo, #fitspiration, and so forth, which promote media that display disordered eating behaviors and idealize thin bodies.[12] Providers can direct families and youths to Web sites and social media channels that are curated by government health organizations (eg, Food and Drug Administration [FDA]; Office of Disease Prevention and Health Promotion; Centers for Disease Control and Prevention), as well as provide education during clinic visits. Identifying social media posts from physicians and health care organizations is more likely to yield unbiased, factual information and helpful advice than posts from individuals or for-profit companies.[13] Increasing adolescents' health literacy by helping them recognize trustworthy sources of information and empowering their families to support them can mitigate potential harm from social media use,[14] and they can connect with people and organizations that promote positive body image and healthy lifestyles.

AMERICAN ACADEMY OF PEDIATRICS CLINICAL PRACTICE GUIDELINES

The American Academy of Pediatrics (AAP) published its first clinical practice guidelines (CPG) for evaluation and treatment of obesity in February 2023.[1] The CPG noted the impact of the pandemic on youths and the need to consider the whole person, family, and the context in which they live, including social determinants of health, when performing an evaluation and developing a treatment plan.[1] While every patient should have intensive health behavior and lifestyle treatment of at least 26 hours in a 3-month to 12-month period, additional treatment can include medication and potentially bariatric surgery, depending on the age, comorbidities, and BMI.[1] The guidelines provide nuances to the recommendations for patients who have class 2 or 3 obesity (class 2: 120% to 140% of the 95th percentile or BMI 35–40 kg/m^2; class 3: $\geq$ 140% of the 95th percentile or BMI $\geq$ 40 kg/m^2).[1]

MOTIVATIONAL INTERVIEWING

To help build a therapeutic relationship, especially considering that weight may be a sensitive topic for many people, it is important to request permission from the patient to discuss it. If permission is granted, asking open-ended questions about their journey, priorities, and concerns can provide insight to guide the conversation. Unfortunately, weight stigma and bias are also present in health care, and the language we use when discussing weight can affect the therapeutic relationship, affecting when and whether patients and families seek health care.[4] Data show that patients often prefer terms such as "weight" and "BMI" over "obese,"[15] and adolescents may prefer "plus size" or "weight problem."[16] The best course of action may be to ask what words they prefer to use, as patients with internalized weight stigma may prefer different language.[4] Motivational interviewing (MI) is a conversation strategy where the goal is to understand the patient's motivations and values, have them express their reasons to do or not do a behavior, and decide the next steps.[17] The provider is a guide, not a judge, and can help frame the patient's goals into a SMART structure: specific, measurable, achievable, relevant, and time-bound. A systematic review and meta-analysis from 2022 explored the effect of MI-based interventions on behavior change in adolescents in weight management programs, and it found that MI helped reduce intake of sugar-sweetened beverages but did not impact BMI or body composition.[18] However, MI can provide a framework for how to approach conversations around weight, focusing on patient autonomy.

EVALUATION

As part of the initial history, providers should ask patients about medications and supplements that are obesogenic.[1] Per the AAP's CPG, laboratory tests for adolescents with obesity should evaluate lipid levels (eg, fasting lipid panel), glucose metabolism (eg, hemoglobin A1c), and liver function (eg, alanine transaminase), and blood pressure should be checked at each visit to screen for hypertension.[1] Further testing could include evaluation for polycystic ovarian syndrome (PCOS) in females with irregular menstrual cycles or evidence of hyperandrogenism on examination.[1] Imaging is guided by the history and physical examination (H&P), for example, obtaining plain radiographs if there is concern for slipped capital femoral epiphysis (SCFE) or Blount disease.[1] A sleep history would guide decisions to refer the patient for a polysomnogram to evaluate for obstructive sleep apnea (OSA).[1] If patients have new or worsening headaches, they should be examined for papilledema and sixth nerve palsy, which are signs of idiopathic intracranial hypertension (IIH).[1] Mental health and eating disorders increased during the COVID-19 pandemic and can impact the treatment of obesity and comorbidities, so patients should be screened for depression, anxiety, and disordered eating behaviors, using validated screening tools such as the Patient Health

Questionnaire for Adolescents (PHQ-A), General Anxiety Disorder-7 (GAD-7), and Eating Attitudes Test-26 (EAT-26).[19–21]

Evaluation Overview

Review medications and supplements, screening for obesogenic drugs.

Check blood pressure at every visit.

Laboratory tests: remember lipids, liver, A1c

H&P: keep in mind PCOS, OSA, IIH, SCFE, Blount disease

Screening: PHQ-A, GAD-7, EAT-26

MANAGEMENT
Goals

The primary goal of the management of obesity is the prevention and remission of comorbidities. Evidence shows that a loss of 5% to 10% of total body weight can improve obesity-related comorbidities,[1] although in some patients, achieving remission may require losing over 10% of one's weight.[22] Weight reduction, particularly after bariatric surgery, can also lead to improved health-related quality of life.[1,22]

Therapeutic Options

In addition to intensive lifestyle interventions, the AAP's CPG recommends adding anti-obesity pharmacotherapy to the care plan for adolescents aged 12 years and older with obesity, based on individual risks, benefits, and patient preference.[1] FDA-approved medications for patients aged 12 years and up with obesity include orlistat, phentermine/topiramate, liraglutide, and semaglutide; phentermine/topiramate and semaglutide were approved in 2022.[23] Other medications are approved for adults with obesity or for those who have a comorbidity (eg, T2DM) and may be used off-label for patients without comorbidities.[1] Bariatric surgery referral may be offered to adolescents with class 2 obesity and significant comorbidities or those with class 3 obesity, even if no comorbidities are present.[1,24] The PCORnet bariatric study from 2018 examined outcomes from bariatric surgeries in adolescents and found that the vertical gastric sleeve and Roux-en-Y gastric bypass procedures yielded greater BMI reduction relative to the adjustable gastric banding surgery[25]; the vertical gastric sleeve procedure is preferred in adolescents.[24]

Outcomes and Complications

Among the medications that are FDA approved for weight loss in adolescents, semaglutide is the most effective at inducing weight loss, and it also improves metabolic parameters.[23] Its dosing schedule and side effect profile are well tolerated by most patients; however, discontinuing the medication leads to weight regain.[23] The combination phentermine/topiramate therapy can increase the risk of suicidal ideation, slow linear growth and cognition, and it can cause congenital defects if taken during the first trimester of pregnancy.[23] Orlistat is uncommonly used in part due to its intolerable gastrointestinal side effects.[1,23]

  For adolescents with severe obesity, bariatric surgery yields an average weight loss of 27% that is sustained for 3 to 5 years or more and leads to remission of comorbidities.[24] Beyond the potential for adverse events in the intraoperative and acute postoperative periods, long-term complications of bariatric surgery can include weight regain, decreased bone density, and vitamin deficiencies.[23] Patients must adhere to particular eating patterns due to the smaller capacity of the stomach and must take life-long vitamin supplementation.[23,24] Adolescents are also at risk of internal hernias,[24] gall stones,[23] and may need additional surgeries to manage excessive loose skin, particularly at the abdomen.[26] Females also need to be counseled for the risk of unplanned pregnancy, as fertility improves with weight loss.[27]

Potential Pitfalls

Shortages

There have been worldwide shortages of semaglutide, particularly after its brand names Wegovy (approved for weight loss) and Ozempic (approved for patients with T2DM) started trending on TikTok in 2022; its effects were lauded by celebrities, making it challenging for patients with T2DM to obtain the medicines.[28] The FDA maintains a database of current drug shortages, and semaglutide has been listed as in shortage for at least 1 formulation since March 2022.[29] As of February 2024, all of the lower dosages of Wegovy are in shortage (all strengths except the maintenance dosage),[29] which limits the ability of prescribers to start patients on the medication. Novo Nordisk, the manufacturer of Wegovy, plans to increase the supply of lower dose formulations by over 100% in 2024.[30]

Cost and insurance coverage

Wegovy has a list price of over $16,000 for a year supply, and Novo Nordisk offers savings plans only for patients with commercial insurance and only for their first 12 prescription fills.[31] Only 9 states include Wegovy on their Medicaid drug formulary,[32] highlighting disparate access to the medication based on income, insurance coverage, and geographic location. Even those with commercial insurance may have difficulty affording the medication after the first year when they are no longer eligible for the manufacturer's discounts.

Backlash after the publication of American Academy of Pediatrics' clinical practice guidelines

While the AAP's CPG notes that BMI is an imperfect measure, some advocates for Health at Every Size principles are concerned that the messages from the CPG will worsen weight stigma, anti-fat bias, and eating disorders.[33,34] There are also concerns about the unknown long-term effects of semaglutide on adolescents.[34] While there is no single best approach to caring for patients with obesity, there are data showing long-term health effects from excess adiposity, so "watchful waiting" is not effective.[1] To help mitigate stigma and bias at an individual level, providers can assess their own biases using tools such as Implicit Association Tests offered through Project Implicit,[35] and recognition of obesity as a chronic disease can also increase empathy toward patients.[4] As previously noted, providers can use validated screening tools to evaluate patients for disordered eating behaviors and mental health concerns, and they should stay up to date with literature on short-term and long-term effects of anti-obesity medications.

CONTINUING EDUCATION

Providers who are interested in making obesity care a focused part of their practice may be interested in obtaining further education. The American Board of Obesity Medicine (ABOM) offers certification to become a "diplomate," although the American Board of Medical Specialties does not acknowledge obesity medicine as a specialty or subspecialty.[36] Physicians become eligible to take the ABOM examination after completing continuing medical education courses or a fellowship program.[36] Providers who are not physicians (nurse practitioner, physician assistant) can obtain certificates from the Obesity Medicine Association, the American Academy of Physicians Associates, and The American Society of Metabolic and Bariatric Surgery.[36]

SUMMARY

This article gives a brief overview of obesity management in the post-pandemic landscape. Considering the potential sensitivity of discussion of weight and body size, it is vital to form a therapeutic relationship with the adolescent and family, guide them toward unbiased forms of media, and use shared decision-making when setting goals and developing a plan of care. Pharmacotherapy options can be effective but must be taken chronically, and insurance coverage for semaglutide is unlikely, especially if taken solely for weight loss without comorbidities. Bariatric surgery is effective long-term and leads to the remission of comorbidities. Health professionals and the community should continue to discuss weight stigma and work to minimize weight bias in health care. Further education is available for physicians through ABOM.

CLINICS CARE POINTS

- Ask permission to discuss weight; be mindful of weight stigma and bias.
- Use MI and shared decision-making to craft SMART goals, engaging the adolescent and caregivers and prioritizing patient autonomy.
- Screen for mental health concerns, disordered eating behaviors, and problematic social media usage.
- Direct patients and families to trustworthy Web sites and social media channels.
- Offer interventions early as opposed to "watchful waiting."
- Behavior management and lifestyle changes are central to every care plan.
- Semaglutide is the most effective FDA-approved medication for weight loss in adolescents but is unlikely to be covered by insurance at this time.
- Bariatric surgery may be an option for adolescents with severe obesity with or without comorbidities.
- Continuing education in obesity medicine is available for physicians and allied health professionals.

DISCLOSURE

Dr A.M. Swamy has no commercial or financial conflicts of interest. No funding sources were provided for this article.

REFERENCES

1. Hampl SE, Hassink SG, Skinner AC, et al. Clinical practice guideline for the evaluation and treatment of children and adolescents with obesity. Pediatrics 2023; 151(2). e2022060640.
2. Iacopetta D, Catalano A, Ceramella J, et al. The Ongoing Impact of COVID-19 on Pediatric Obesity. Pediatr Rep 2024;16(1):135–50.
3. Nogueira-de-Almeida CA, Del Ciampo LA, Ferraz IS, et al. COVID-19 and obesity in childhood and adolescence: a clinical review. J Pediatr 2020;96(5):546–58.

4. Haqq AM, Kebbe M, Tan Q, et al. Complexity and stigma of pediatric obesity. Child Obes 2021;17(4):229–40.
5. Goettler A, Grosse A, Sonntag D. Productivity loss due to overweight and obesity: a systematic review of indirect costs. BMJ Open 2017;7(10):e014632.
6. Fryar CD, Carroll MD, Afful J. Prevalence of overweight, obesity, and severe obesity among children and adolescents aged 2–19 years: United States, 1963–1965 through 2017–2018. NCHS Health E-Stats 2020.
7. Woolford SJ, Sidell M, Li X, et al. Changes in body mass index among children and adolescents during the COVID-19 Pandemic. JAMA 2021;326(14):1434–6.
8. Dunton GF, Do B, Wang SD. Early effects of the COVID-19 pandemic on physical activity and sedentary behavior in children living in the U.S. BMC Publ Health 2020;20(1):1351.
9. Pietrobelli A, Pecoraro L, Ferruzzi A, et al. Effects of COVID-19 lockdown on life-style behaviors in children with obesity living in verona, italy: a longitudinal study. Obesity (Silver Spring) 2020;28(8):1382–5.
10. Adams EL, Caccavale LJ, Smith D, et al. Food insecurity, the home food environment, and parent feeding practices in the era of COVID-19. Obesity (Silver Spring) 2020;28(11):2056–63.
11. Puhl RM. Weight stigma, policy initiatives, and harnessing social media to elevate activism. Body Image 2022;40:131–7.
12. Jebeile H, Partridge SR, Gow ML, et al. Adolescent exposure to weight loss imagery on instagram: a content analysis of "top" images. Child Obes 2021;17(4):241–8.
13. Aiman U, Mylavarapu M, Gohil NV, et al. Obesity: an instagram analysis. Cureus 2023;15(5):e39619.
14. Lahti H, Kulmala M, Hietajärvi L, et al. What counteracts problematic social media use in adolescence? a cross-national observational study. J Adolesc Health 2024; 74(1):98–112.
15. Auckburally S, Davies E, Logue J. The use of effective language and communication in the management of obesity: the challenge for healthcare professionals. Curr Obes Rep 2021;10(3):274–81.
16. Puhl RM, Himmelstein MS. Adolescent preferences for weight terminology used by health care providers. Pediatr Obes 2018;13(9):533–40.
17. Rollnick S, Miller WR. What is motivational interviewing? Behav Cognit Psychother 1995;23(4):325–34.
18. Amiri P, Mansouri-Tehrani MM, Khalili-Chelik A, et al. Does motivational interviewing improve the weight management process in adolescents? a systematic review and meta-analysis. Int J Behav Med 2022;29(1):78–103.
19. Lin JA, Hartman-Munick SM, Kells MR, et al. The impact of the COVID-19 pandemic on the number of adolescents/young adults seeking eating disorder-related care. J Adolesc Health 2021;69(4):660–3.
20. Panchal U, Salazar de Pablo G, Franco M, et al. The impact of COVID-19 lockdown on child and adolescent mental health: systematic review. Eur Child Adolesc Psychiatr 2023;32(7):1151–77.
21. Solmi F, Downs JL, Nicholls DE. COVID-19 and eating disorders in young people. Lancet Child Adolesc Health 2021;5(5):316–8.
22. Tahrani AA, Morton J. Benefits of weight loss of 10% or more in patients with overweight or obesity: A review. Obesity (Silver Spring) 2022;30(4):802–40.
23. Vajravelu ME, Tas E, Arslanian S. Pediatric obesity: complications and current day management. Life 2023;13(7):1591.

24. Singhal V, Youssef S, Misra M. Use of sleeve gastrectomy in adolescents and young adults with severe obesity. Curr Opin Pediatr 2020;32(4):547–53.
25. Inge TH, Coley RY, Bazzano LA, et al. Comparative effectiveness of bariatric procedures among adolescents: the PCORnet bariatric study. Surg Obes Relat Dis 2018;14(9):1374–86.
26. Derderian SC, Dewberry LC, Patten L, et al. Excess skin problems among adolescents after bariatric surgery. Surg Obes Relat Dis 2020;16(8):993–8.
27. Cena H, Chiovato L, Nappi RE. Obesity, polycystic ovary syndrome, and infertility: a new avenue for GLP-1 receptor agonists. J Clin Endocrinol Metab 2020; 105(8):e2695–709.
28. Daignault M. Elon Musk's weight loss, Ozempic, Wegovy and what to know about the new TikTok viral treatment. USA Today. 2022. Available at: https://www.usatoday.com/story/life/health-wellness/2022/10/20/ozempic-weight-loss-wegovy-what-know-diabetes-injections-tiktok/10538361002/. [Accessed 1 October 2023].
29. U.S. Food and Drug Administration. Current and Resolved Drug Shortages and Discontinuations Reported to FDA. Available at: https://www.accessdata.fda.gov/scripts/drugshortages/default.cfm. [Accessed 26 February 2024].
30. Novo Nordisk. Updates About Wegovy®. Available at: https://www.novonordisk-us.com/supply-update.html. [Accessed 26 February 2024].
31. Novo Nordisk. Save on Wegovy®. Available at: https://www.wegovy.com/coverage-and-savings/save-on-wegovy.html. [Accessed 26 February 2024].
32. Belloni G. Next-gen weight-loss drugs receive tentative embrace by medicaid. In: Bloomberg Law. 2023. Available at: https://news.bloomberglaw.com/health-law-and-business/next-gen-weight-loss-drugs-receive-tentative-embrace-by-medicaid. [Accessed 26 February 2024].
33. Association for Size Diversity and Health. ASDAH Opposes the New AAP Ob*sity Guidelines. ASDAH, February 9, 2023. Available at: ashad.org/aapstatement. Accessed October 1, 2023.
34. Dennis K. A Critical Look at New Guidelines for Kids With Higher BMIs. Psychol Today 2023. Available at: https://www.psychologytoday.com/us/blog/live-free/202302/a-critical-look-at-new-guidelines-for-kids-with-higher-bmis. [Accessed 1 October 2023].
35. Project Implicit. Available at: https://implicit.harvard.edu/implicit/takeatest.html.
36. Fitch A, Horn DB, Still CD, et al. Obesity medicine as a subspecialty and United States certification - A review. Obesity Pillars 2023;(6):100062.

Impact of the COVID-19 Pandemic on Youth Substance Use and Substance-Related Risk Factors and Outcomes

Implications for Prevention, Treatment, and Policy

Christopher J. Hammond, MD, PhD[a,b,*], Kathryn Van Eck, PhD[b,c], Hoover Adger, MD, MPH, MBA[b]

KEYWORDS

- Youth substance use • Youth substance use disorders • COVID-19 pandemic
- Risk factors • Vulnerable subgroups • Substance use treatment

KEY POINTS

- COVID-19 pandemic had a significant impact on daily life for young people globally and produced complex and, at times, opposing effects on risk and protective factors for addictive disorders.
- The prevalence rates of substance use decreased among adolescents in the general US population during the COVID-19 pandemic.
- Overdoses and overdose deaths increased significantly among US youth during the COVID-19 pandemic as a result of unintentional and intentional fentanyl exposure.
- The impact of the COVID-19 pandemic on adolescent substance use varied as a function of prepandemic and during pandemic risk factors, with use rates increasing in some vulnerable subgroups.
- The impact of partial clinic closures and shift to telehealth and hybrid treatment formats for substance use disorder treatment in youth remains unclear, but may have worsened disparities for vulnerable youth and families.

[a] Division of Child & Adolescent Psychiatry, Department of Psychiatry, Johns Hopkins University School of Medicine, Johns Hopkins Bayview, 5500 Lombard Street, Baltimore, MD 21224, USA; [b] Division of Adolescent & Young Adult Medicine, Department of Pediatrics, Johns Hopkins University School of Medicine, 200 North Wolfe Street, Baltimore, MD 21287, USA; [c] Kennedy Krieger Institute, 1741 Ashland Avenue, Baltimore, MD 21205, USA
* Corresponding author. Johns Hopkins Bayview, 5500 Lombard Street, Baltimore, MD 21224.
E-mail address: chammo20@jhmi.edu

Pediatr Clin N Am 71 (2024) 653–669
https://doi.org/10.1016/j.pcl.2024.05.002   **pediatric.theclinics.com**

INTRODUCTION

Adolescence is a critical developmental period marked by significant biological, psychological, and behavioral changes that include pubertal maturation, identity formation, and increased exploratory behaviors and peer socialization.[1] Within this biobehavioral developmental stage and ecological context, adolescent substance use and substance use disorders (SUDs) are common and represent an ongoing public health issue in the United States.[2] Adolescent substance use, particularly regular use, is associated with adverse psychosocial and health outcomes, including unintentional injuries, suicide, aggression, motor vehicle crashes, academic and vocational failure, sexually transmitted infections, unintended pregnancy, and increased risk for developing psychiatric disorders and SUD by young adulthood.[3–6]

Youth substance use and SUD are best conceptualized as "pediatric-onset" developmental disorders that show intergenerational transmission.[7] Most individuals who develop lifetime SUD report that they started using alcohol/drugs regularly before age 18 years. Substance initiation, progression to regular use, and initial age of onset of SUD diagnoses peak during adolescence and young adulthood.[8] There are known childhood-onset risk and protective factors at the level of the individual, family, and community that influence the likelihood that an adolescent will start using alcohol/drugs and develop an SUD.[9] These factors can be targeted as part of substance use prevention interventions. Given the emerging evidence for developmental sensitivity and negative effect on downstream health outcomes related to substance exposure, studies examining how environmental factors, such as major global events, impact youth substance use and SUD outcomes are needed and can inform development of prevention and early intervention strategies.

The COVID-19 pandemic represents one of the most impactful events affecting the daily lives and health behaviors for youth of this generation. On March 11, 2020, the World Health Organization declared the coronavirus SARS-CoV-2 (COVID-19) a pandemic.[10] Over the ensuing 3 years, more than 400 million cases and nearly 6 million deaths worldwide have been attributed to COVID-19.[11] In an effort to stop the spread of the virus, the federal, state, and local municipalities across the United States and globally enacted various laws including lockdowns, curfews, border closures, stay-at-home orders, mandated social distancing, masking requirements, closing of schools and shifting to remote learning, stopping extracurricular and sports programs and other youth services, prohibition of social gatherings, and restricting access to worksites and entertainment venues.[12,13] The pandemic and pandemic-related risk mitigation efforts have resulted in unintended downstream consequences for youth, which are still being experienced. School closings and shifts to remote learning have impacted student learning and resulted in school-aged children falling behind academically compared to prior cohorts, with these deficits being more impactful for low-income and minoritized youth, exacerbating preexisting educational inequalities. The loss of work and income for caregivers has placed financial strain on parents/caregivers and families. Lockdowns, curfews, stay-at-home orders, and restrictions on social gathering increased feelings of loneliness among young people during the pandemic.[14,15] Additionally, adolescents experienced increased rates of depression, anxiety, and suicidal ideations during the pandemic,[16] all of which are risk factors for early-onset substance use and SUD. At the same time, social distancing and lockdown measures may have disrupted drug using peer networks and decreased access for youth.[17] How these directionally opposing effects on substance-related risk and protective factors have impacted youth and contributed to changes in youth substance use remains poorly understood.

In this article, we examine the impact of the COVID-19 pandemic on substance use behaviors and SUD outcomes for US youth, with a focus on characterizing vulnerable subgroups and identifying factors that contribute to variance in these outcomes. We discuss prepandemic and during pandemic individual- and environmental-level factors associated with increased and decreased substance use and SUD outcomes in adolescents during the pandemic. Finally, we review implications for treatment, prevention, policy, and future research.

EFFECTS OF COVID-19 PANDEMIC ON YOUTH SUBSTANCE USE

Alcohol and other drug use among adolescents was common prior to the pandemic, although rates had been decreasing for many substances (excluding cannabis) even prior to this event.[18] Perhaps the best data on pandemic-related changes in youth substance use can be drawn from national survey data. For example, data on current and prepandemic substance use rates from the Monitoring the Future (MTF) survey, a national cross-sectional survey administered annually to middle and high school students across the United States, can provide insight into changing trends in use during this time period (**Table 1**).[18,19] In 2022, among US 12th graders, 51.9% reported past-year alcohol use, 30.7% reported past-year cannabis use, and 8.0% reported past-year illicit drug use other than cannabis (eg, cocaine, heroin, methamphetamine).[20] Tobacco product use, particularly related to nicotine vaping, is also common with 27.3% of US 12th graders reporting past-year use. Prepandemic prevalence data on past-year alcohol use, cannabis use, non-cannabis illicit drug use, and tobacco/nicotine vaping among US 12th graders from the 2019 MTF survey were 52.1%, 35.7%, 11.5%, and 35.3% respectively.[21] Focusing on trends in use across age groups, as shown in **Table 1**, past-year prevalence rates for alcohol use, cannabis use, illicit drug use other than cannabis, and tobacco vaping all decreased among US 8th, 10th, and 12th graders during the pandemic. Of note, past-year substance use prevalence rates reached all-time lows across drug categories in 2021 but then rose in 2022, suggesting that this shift may have been temporary.[21] For example, while remaining below prepandemic levels, annual rates of alcohol use and cannabis use both increased significantly in 2022. Continued surveillance of substance use trends is important.

Studies examining the effects of the COVID-19 pandemic can shed additional light on pandemic-related changes in youth substance use but have shown inconsistent results, with some studies showing increased use and others showing decreased use or no change in substance use during the pandemic.[22–29] Some of this variability may be the result of different responses to the pandemic among different subgroups of youth with different prepandemic factors or who experienced more pandemic-related adversities[30] and variation in the patterns of change across different drug categories.[31] Variation in study outcomes may also be related to differences in study design, analytical strategy, sampling frame, study population, outcomes measured, and time period assessed. Many studies used convenience samples and online survey methods to query youth substance use during the pandemic. It is also important to note that all studies identified in our review relied on youth self-report of substance use, and none included biochemical assays of substance use outcomes.

Based on the large number of studies, it is beyond the scope of this article to cover all pandemic-related reports. As such, our review and analysis focus on summative results and specific exemplary studies. One online survey of Canadian adolescents (*n* = 1084, 14–18 year olds) examined changes in self-reported substance use from 3 weeks before to 3 weeks after the start of the pandemic.[32] Results from this study

Table 1
Past-year use of substances of different types in combined sample of US 8th, 10th, and 12th graders from 2019 to 2022 showing pandemic and post-pandemic-related changes

Substance Type	2019	2020	2021	2022	2019–2021 Change[d]	2021–2022 Change[e]
Alcohol	35.9	38.2	30.2	32.2	−5.7[c]	+2.0[b]
Cannabis	25.2	24.9	17.9	19.4	−7.3[c]	+1.5[a]
Any illicit drug other than cannabis	9.0	9.2	5.6	6.1	−3.4[c]	+0.5
Nonmedical prescription opioids[f]	2.7	2.3	1.5	2.1	−1.2	+0.6
Nonmedical prescription stimulants[g]	4.0	4.3	2.2	3.7	−1.8[c]	+1.5[c]
Hallucinogens	2.9	3.4	2.4	2.5	−0.5	+0.1
Cocaine	1.4	1.4	0.7	0.7	−0.7[b]	+0.0
Heroin	0.3	0.2	0.2	0.3	−0.1	+0.1[a]
Methamphetamine	0.5	0.7	0.2	0.3	−0.3[b]	+0.2[a]
Vaping nicotine	27.3	27.1	19.2	19.7	−8.1[c]	+0.5
Vaping cannabis	15.6	16.3	11.6	13.6	−4.0[b]	+2.0[a]

Note: Source of the results are from the Monitoring the Future study, 2023 the University of Michigan.[21] Numbers represent the percentage of combined sample of US 8th, 10th, and 12th graders responding "yes" to question about past-year use of different types of substances for each year. Change numbers represent absolute change in percentage of sample responding "yes" to questions about past-year use of different types of substances from 2019 to 2021 and from 2021 to 2022, respectively. Statistical significance of change rates denoted by the following:
  [a] $P < .05$.
  [b] $P < .01$.
  [c] $P < .001$.
  [d] Changes in past-year substance use from 2019 to 2021 represent change from prepandemic (2019) through the first 2 years of the pandemic (2020 and 2021).
  [e] Changes in past-year substance use from 2021 to 2022 represents change from second year of pandemic (2021) to post-pandemic period (2022).
  [f] Nonmedical prescription opioids = Combined annual rates of oxycodone and vicodin misuse.
  [g] Nonmedical prescription stimulants = Combined annual rates of adderall and ritalin misuse.

showed that youth in the total sample showed a reduction in binge drinking, vaping, and cannabis use, but not alcohol use during the pandemic. Adolescents in the sample who did use substances showed an increase in frequency in use for alcohol and cannabis during the first 3 weeks of the pandemic. Another recent study showed a similar distinction between groups that varied based on their substance use patterns. Gohari and colleagues used latent transition analyses to identify prepandemic patterns of alcohol use in a large sample of Canadian high school students and then examined during pandemic drinking patterns in these groups.[33] They found that low-frequency drinkers and younger students were more likely to reduce their drinking and binge drinking during the pandemic compared to more established drinkers. Pelham and colleagues conducted one of the largest longitudinal studies to examine COVID-19-related changes in adolescent substance use to date, using data on self-reported substance use from 7842 early adolescents from the Adolescent Brain Cognition and Development study cohort.[31] Results from this study showed that the COVID-19 pandemic was associated with a reduction in alcohol use and an increase in the use of nicotine and misuse of prescription drugs among early adolescents. It also showed that in general, rates of early adolescent substance use during the first 6 months of the pandemic remained stable, and mostly reflected low-level episodic use.

With the growing number of studies in this space, a focus on summative results is warranted. Layman and colleagues recently conducted a systematic review of changes in substance use among youth (ages 12–24 years) during the pandemic and identified 49 studies examining changes in prevalence rates of substance use across alcohol (32 studies), cannabis (20 studies), cigarette smoking (27 studies), nicotine vaping (16 studies), and other drug use or unspecified general drug use (19 studies).[34] In their review and analysis, the investigators found that the majority of the studies across drug categories showed a reduction in the prevalence of substance use among general populations of youth, although results were less consistent for studies focused on other and illicit drug use.

Beyond use rates, there is also evidence for a change in the patterns and contexts of substance use and in substance-related adverse outcomes among US adolescents during the COVID-19 pandemic.[18,35] One study focusing on changes in patterns/contexts of use found that most adolescent substance use occurred alone (49%) followed by with parents (42%), with friends using technology (32%), and in-person with friends (24%).[32] This use of alcohol/drugs alone is notable and concerning, given studies showing that using alone is associated with poorer mental health outcomes and higher risk for overdose deaths.[36] The study's finding that many youth used substances with their parents during the pandemic (42% used with parents, 26% binge drank with parents), highlights the need for improved parent/caregiver and family-focused education and prevention efforts for at-risk youth. This is particularly important, as parent permissibility, modeling of parent substance use behaviors, and early-onset substance use represent major risk factors for future substance use and the development of SUD.[37,38] Related to this point, adult substance use and parent alcohol permissibility both increased during the pandemic, with one study showing that during the first 3 months of the pandemic nearly 1 in 6 parents of early adolescents newly allowed their child to drink at home.[39]

During the pandemic, the number of unintentional drug overdoses and overdose deaths in 12 to 24 year olds has risen sharply. National mortality data show that rates of drug overdose deaths among US adolescents increased more than 2.3 fold in the 4 year time period between 2019 and 2021, reaching record highs of 5.49 deaths per 100,000 youth in 2021.[40] According to the US Center for Disease Control and Prevention (CDC), monthly overdose deaths nearly tripled among 10 to 19 year olds during the first 2 years of the COVID-19 pandemic, increasing from an average of 31 to 87 deaths per month from July 2019 to May 2023 before declining to 51 deaths per month in December 2021.[41] These deaths are predominantly related to an increased fentanyl exposure in context of widespread expansion of illicitly manufactured fentanyl throughout the US drug supply during the pandemic.[42,43] For example, fentanyl was identified in 77.1% of overdose deaths compared to benzodiazepines and prescription opioids which were identified in 13.3% and 5.8%, respectively.[40] Underrepresented youth are disproportionately affected by this evolving fentanyl-centric opioid overdose crisis. Recent data indicate that Black youth ages 15 to 24 years had among the highest drug overdose death rates and experienced the largest rate of increase (86%) in overdose deaths during the pandemic, compared to other age and racial groups.[44] The rise in overdose deaths is surprising, in part, as it has occurred concurrently with a reduction in substance use, across categories, in the general population of US youth[20] (although see Pelham and colleagues to the contrary). Many youth overdoses are occurring within the context of unintentional fentanyl exposure by adolescents who are using counterfeit prescription pills adulterated with fentanyl. A number of cases have described early adolescents with no known history of opioid misuse and limited SUD criteria, taking counterfeit prescription pills that they believed to be an amphetamine or benzodiazepine and dying from a fentanyl overdose.[45] The emergence of fentanyl contamination of the US drug supply during the pandemic has shifted the risk level for overdose related to prescription drug misuse and illicit drug use.[42] This shifting risk scale presents a unique challenge to pediatric providers with major implications for clinical practice related to screening, overdose response planning, and prevention.

In summary, the COVID-19 pandemic exerted differential effects on risk and protective factors and has been associated with reductions in the prevalence of substance use across drug categories and increase in overdose deaths among the general population of US adolescents.

FACTORS ASSOCIATED WITH INCREASED YOUTH SUBSTANCE USE DURING COVID-19 PANDEMIC
Prepandemic and During Pandemic Individual-Level Factors Associated with Youth Substance Use

Young adults and adolescents are a demographic at particularly high risk of adverse outcomes of substance use including SUD, and there is a range of factors that influence this. Adolescence is an important stage of human development, and a vital time for laying the foundations of good health.[46] It is also a stage encompassing significant experiences of change and exploration during which risks to health, such as drug and alcohol misuse, may emerge leading to adverse impacts to health and well-being.[47] Adolescent inclination to experiment, peer pressure, challenge rules and authority, and experience low self-worth can also reinforce susceptibility to substance misuse.[48] Factors associated with heightened risk of substance misuse include individual factors such as coexisting mental health disorders, especially depression and anxiety.[49] Broader community and social factors such as peer influence, substance use by a family member, and other family problems can also amplify frequency, amount, and impact of substance use.[50] Further, adolescents involved in either school or cyber bullying (victims, perpetrators, and bully–victims) are also at significantly higher risk of alcohol and substance use.[51]

The use and misuse of alcohol and other drugs remains a leading cause of burden of disease in the adolescent population and can significantly impact acute and long-term morbidity and mortality.[52] The developing adolescent brain is particularly vulnerable to damage from substance use,[53] which may negatively affect development of critical thinking and cognitive skills.[54,55] Substance use/misuse can lead to higher rates of physical and mental health problems and poorer overall health and well-being,[56] psychological distress,[57] school absenteeism and lower grades,[58] increased risk of SUD later in life,[59] decreased help-seeking behavior,[60] and police contact associated with increased mortality and morbidity.[61]

Subgroups of youth at elevated risk for poorer substance-related outcomes during the COVID-19 pandemic

While racially and ethnically underrepresented populations use substances at rates similar to White individuals, underrepresented populations have been and are more likely to experience more severe consequences of their substance use. Compared to their White counterparts, Black, Latinx, and American Indian/Alaska Native populations experience greater mortality rates from substance use, greater severity of SUDs, and increased vulnerability to criminal justice system involvement. Black and Latinx populations, in particular, have more significant barriers accessing and completing substance use treatment and fewer underrepresented adolescents report satisfactory experiences within substance use treatment than White adolescents. These disparities are driven by long-existing intersectional racism and drug-related stigma. Structural racism is manifested in unequal enforcement of drug laws, lower access to evidence-based treatments, and greater odds of experiencing adverse substance-related health outcomes among underrepresented populations. Structural violence is expressed through stigma enacted against people with SUDs and through policies that disqualify people with substance use histories from access to public services, employment, education, and housing. These policies contribute to the poor outcomes and health disparities seen among underrepresented populations with SUDs.

Underrepresented populations experience discrimination at every stage of the judicial system and are more likely to be stopped, searched, arrested, convicted, harshly sentenced and/or burdened with a lifelong criminal record. This is particularly the case for drug law violations, where Black people comprise 29% and 40% of individuals arrested and incarcerated for drug law violations, respectively, despite representing only 13% of the US population and using drugs at similar rates to people of other races. With less than 5% of the world's population, but nearly 25% of its incarcerated population, the US imprisons more people than any other nation in the world. Racialized drug policies with harsh and disparate sentencing requirements have led to profoundly unequal criminal justice outcomes for underrepresented populations with SUDs. Although rates of drug use and sales are similar across racial and ethnic lines, Black and Latinx adolescents are far more likely to have criminal justice involvement and experience stricter consequences compared to White adolescents.

Moreover, gender nonbinary or gender diverse youths experience disproportionately higher rates of substance use, homelessness, mental health concerns, and suicidality. LGBTQIA+ (lesbian, gay, bisexual, transgender, queer, intersex, asexual) communities experienced worse mental health and problem drinking than their cisgender, heteronormative counterparts during the COVID-19 pandemic.[62] Policymakers should consider resources to support LGBTQIA+ mental health and substance use prevention in COVID-19 recovery efforts.[63] Health professionals need to recognize the impact of intersectional stigma and discrimination in these and other vulnerable populations and create intervention and treatment systems that are sensitive to their needs.

Prepandemic and During Pandemic Environmental and Family Factors Associated with Youth Substance Use

The pandemic produced complex and, at times, opposing effects on different addiction-related risk and protective factors that may have produced a net negative protective effect in general and a net risk promoting effect for certain vulnerable subgroups.

COVID-19 created a "perfect storm" in which adolescents and young adults were negatively impacted by an ensuing combination of social, economic and health impacts globally. Forced closure of business, schooling from home, and lockdowns were the hallmarks of the COVID response, and the impact on younger people was acute. Part-time workers were among the most heavily affected, of which younger adults tend to make up a significant proportion. In the United States, the unemployment rates of young workers aged 16 to 24 years jumped from 8.4% in early 2019 to 24.4% a year later.[64] It is not surprising to find that increasing rates of unemployment, financial stress, and a lack of social connection combined to produce worsening mental health for younger people, with this age group reporting symptoms of anxiety or depression at rates 30% to 80% higher than other adults.[65] Moreover, the usual places for mental health support for younger adults and adolescents, namely schools, universities, and workplaces, were largely closed during the COVID-related lockdowns, thereby separating younger people from these protective factors and creating conditions which may contribute to an individual's susceptibility to drug and alcohol use.[32–66] It is interesting to note that places of potential support, particularly schools, have also traditionally been places of peer influence that can increase drug or alcohol use.[17] It may have been possible that separation from these peer influences could have reduced drug and alcohol misuse. Likewise, more time spent at home under parental supervision, with less opportunity for impulsivity and less access to suppliers of drugs and alcohol, might also have limited drug and alcohol misuse and the onset of behaviors that lead to addiction.[17] Yet, the experiences of social isolation, in addition to other factors such as drug and alcohol use by parents in the home, can and did increase substance use in adolescents and young adults.[67] Increases in drug and alcohol misuse, triggered by depression and anxiety and disruption of routines during the COVID-19 pandemic, created an "epidemic hidden in a pandemic."[68]

CHANGES IN SUBSTANCE USE DISORDER TREATMENT AND MENTAL HEALTH POLICY DURING AND POST-COVID-19 PANDEMIC
What Youth Need for Effective Substance Use Prevention and Substance Use Disorder Treatment

Responses to the increase in the mental health and substance use-related problems need to come from multiple levels and help to build upon known protective factors including: promoting optimism; teaching mindfulness; strengthening beliefs regarding accurate substance use norms, supporting the desire to maintain one's health; enhancing parental engagement in the lives of adolescents and their awareness of the harms of drug use behaviors; enhancing school connectedness; supporting structured prosocial activities in our communities; and supporting strong religious beliefs.[69]

At the individual level, interventions predominantly focus on reducing consumption in adolescents based on the principles of motivational interviewing, acknowledging adolescents and young adult's values and strengths, and strengthening acknowledgment of the inherent worth and potential of our youth.[70] All of these can be promoted by the health care professional in their interactions with adolescents and young adults.

Family-based interventions highlight that the family context has huge effects on the development of children and adolescents.[71] The family can have direct and indirect impacts on the occurrence of substance use and SUD and is fundamental to effective interventions.[50–72] Family-based approaches to intervention and treatment are often more effective than individual approaches alone as they may improve not just substance use/SUD of affected youth but also family functioning.[73] Health professionals can facilitate interventions aimed at the family level by prioritizing enhancement of family function and acknowledging the important role of the family in effecting change.[50]

Schools are a key source for intervention programs given their central role in the life and social connectedness of adolescents and some young adults. School-based programs can bring together different approaches in multidimensional programs and have the potential to prevent, delay onset, and reduce the prevalence and effect of substance use in the population.[74] Close networks with peers can influence adolescents' health behaviors and social environments, reducing their risk and working instead as a protective factor against substance use and the progression to SUD.[75]

At the patient care and clinical level, health care professionals can assist with reversing the effects of COVID-19 isolation and social disconnection in adolescents and young adults through acknowledgment of the link between mental health and substance use. A key driver of increased substance use and related problems is poor mental health triggered by social, economic, and psychological impacts of COVID-19 and a key avenue to counter this increase lies in creating better mental health supports. Good mental health can be promoted and preserved through multifaceted, overlaying of approaches to better health that focus on better sleep, nutrition, exercise, family functioning, resilience, and social and educational functioning.

COVID-19 Pandemic-Related Changes in Substance Use Treatment and Health Policy

An unfortunate and sad reality of the day is the finding from multiple studies which show that youth who are in need of prevention, early intervention, and treatment are less able to access treatment of SUD compared to adults, and the treatment options offered to youth are substantially different and limited compared to those offered to adults.[76] Among youth who experienced a nonfatal opioid overdose, only 2% received pharmacotherapy within 30 days of overdosing and 29% received behavioral health services alone; more than 70% received no addiction treatment.[77] Behavioral interventions without medication are the mainstay for treatment of SUD among youth, despite guidelines recommending the use of pharmacotherapy in young patients.[78,79]

Although there exist national resources offering pediatric-focused training and support, as well as a wealth of policy statements, clinical reports, and educational materials, there still seems to be a paucity of pediatric addiction medicine subspecialists and there are few youth-focused providers (ie, child and adolescent psychiatrists, pediatricians, and adolescent medicine physicians) who are able to prescribe pharmacotherapy for SUDs, and fewer who are willing to, or have experience, prescribing other medications shown to improve outcomes for SUDs.[80,81] While there is a need to address and rectify the dearth of trained youth-focused physicians, there have been some changes in the field to address some of the challenges in medical management for patient with SUDs and add to the armamentarium and tools and help to address some of the barriers.

The US government introduced several policies during the COVID-19 pandemic that aimed to facilitate access to opioid use disorder (OUD) treatment. Some policies are temporary in nature, including those tied to the public health emergency (PHE) declaration for COVID-19, while others are permanent.

Federal regulations for opiate treatment programs (OTPs) in the US have historically restricted the dispensing of methadone doses for unsupervised ("take-home") use based on the length of time a patient has been receiving comprehensive treatment (eg, during the first 90 days of treatment the take-home supply is limited to a single dose each week), while at the same time giving individual OTPs the discretion to make case-by-case determinations about take-home supply (within these time-in-treatment regulatory parameters) for individual patients guided by clinical stability and risk (ie, substance abstinence, regular clinic attendance, and stability). As a result of these regulations, many individuals were typically required to visit an OTP daily to receive their dose. In response to the COVID-19 pandemic, the US substance abuse and mental health services administration (SAMHSA) permitted states to request blanket exceptions to time-in-treatment requirements in order to minimize the risk of COVID-19 transmission at OTPs and preserve the supply of personal protective equipment.[82] These exceptions allowed OTPs to dispense up to 28 days of take-home methadone doses to "stable" patients and up to 14 days of take-home doses for "less stable" patients. Forty-three states and the District of Columbia received exceptions during the pandemic. In November 2021, SAMHSA announced that it was extending the modified take-home dose standards for 1 year beyond the eventual expiration of the COVID-19 PHE declaration, while it pursues rulemaking to make these flexibilities permanent.[83] For the duration of the COVID-19 PHE, the US drug enforcement agency (DEA) also eased several OTP requirements to mitigate potential disruptions to treatment. Under these relaxed standards, OTP clinical staff, other authorized OTP staff, law enforcement officers, and National Guard members are permitted to make doorstep deliveries of methadone and buprenorphine to clients undergoing quarantine or isolation due to COVID-19.[84] The DEA has also allowed OTPs to repeatedly use the same off-site location to dispense methadone and buprenorphine without separately registering the location, subject to certain requirements.[85–88] Additionally, in June 2021, the DEA permanently eliminated a moratorium on approving mobile components of OTPs (eg, vans) and waived separate registration requirements.[89]

Telehealth-based addiction services during COVID-19 pandemic
Historically, practitioners must conduct at least one in-person medical evaluation with a patient prior to issuing a prescription for a controlled substance via telehealth, with several exceptions. The US department of health and human services (HHS) and department of justice (DOJ) exercised one exception for the COVID-19 PHE, which allows the prescribing of controlled substances via telehealth using a real-time, 2 way, audiovisual communication device without having an initial in-person visit.[90] For the prescribing of buprenorphine for OUD, the DEA further relaxed requirements by allowing the use of audio-only devices (eg, telephone).[91]

SAMHSA has similarly allowed OTPs to initiate treatment with buprenorphine after a telehealth visit and continues treating existing patients with buprenorphine or methadone via telehealth (using either audiovisual or audio-only devices). Additionally, the Centers for Medicare & Medicaid Services has modified Medicare coverage requirements during the COVID-19 PHE to allow the therapy and counseling components of OTP services to be conducted via telehealth (including use of audio-only devices).[92]

Buprenorphine waiver requirements changed during the COVID-19 pandemic
The process to obtain a waiver to prescribe buprenorphine has traditionally involved completing training (with some exceptions) and submitting a notice of intent to SAMHSA, in which a practitioner certifies their capacity to provide or refer patients to counseling and other ancillary services.[93] Recent legislative changes remove the federal requirement to submit a notice of intent to prescribe medications such as buprenorphine for opioid use disorder. All practitioners who have a current DEA registration that includes Schedule III authority may now prescribe buprenorphine for opioid use disorder as permitted by applicable state law. In addition, there is no longer a cap on the number of patients that a practitioner can treat.

FUTURE DIRECTIONS FOR CLINICAL PRACTICE AND RESEARCH

Based on the information described earlier related to the effects of COVID-19 pandemic on youth substance use, future directions for practice and research should include

- Integrating routine screening for substance use and SUD within the pediatric primary care setting through the evidence-based tools and skills that leverage youth strengths, such as motivational interviewing. Pediatric health professionals must receive ongoing training not only in how to recognize and treat substance use and SUD in primary care settings but also in how to recognize the role of their own implicit and explicit biases in treatment discussions.

- Making it standard that treatment programs disseminate information on race and ethnicity, as well as outcome metrics, to better identify the programs most effective at addressing the needs of minoritized youths.
- Expanding access to evidence-based interventions and therapies for youth, including state-of-the-art therapeutics and medications offered in specialty addiction treatment settings and in primary care settings serving youth.
- Developing and testing the efficacy of treatment programs that are tailored to the developmental needs of youth and that address the impact of racial and other types of structural violence on well-being.
- Supporting positive youth development and behavioral models of care that respond to the unique circumstances of youths with SUD and recognize the role that the direct effects of racism or discrimination may have on youth well-being.

SUMMARY

In conclusion, the COVID-19 pandemic has had complex effects on substance use behaviors and outcomes among youth that vary based on prepandemic and during pandemic factors. Collective results from national survey data and pandemic-specific studies show that the prevalence rates of substance use decreased during the pandemic and may be rising in this post-pandemic period. At the same time, the rates of overdoses and overdose deaths among US adolescents related to fentanyl have increased sharply during the pandemic reflecting a more dangerous illicit US drug supply. Findings during the COVID-19 pandemic highlight the need for parental education on adolescent substance use and family-based interventions for adolescents engaged in substance use. Adolescent mental health, a significant driver of substance use behavior, was substantially impacted by social, economic, and psychological impacts of COVID-19, demonstrating additional domains where implementing equitable approaches may have meaningful preventive effects on adolescent substance use. Finally, there is a significant need for culturally responsive intervention adaptation and development to address the intersectional experiences and challenges of underrepresented youth.

CLINICS CARE POINTS

- Need for integration of routine screening for substance use and SUD within the pediatric primary care setting through evidence-based tools and skills that leverage youth strengths, such as motivational interviewing.

- Pediatric health professionals need ongoing training not only in how to recognize and treat substance use and SUD in primary care settings but also in how to recognize the role of their own implicit and explicit biases in treatment discussions.

- Pediatricians should attempt to create a confidential space for check-ins during clinical encounters and routinely review the limits of confidentiality with adolescents.

- Expanded access to evidence-based interventions and therapies for youth, including state-of-the-art therapeutics and medications offered in specialty addiction treatment settings and primary care settings serving youth is needed.

- Next steps include developing and testing the efficacy of treatment programs that are tailored to the developmental needs of youth and that address the impact of racial and other types of structural violence on well-being.

• Supporting positive youth development and behavioral models of care that respond to the unique circumstances of youths with SUD and recognize the role that the direct effects of racism or discrimination may have on youth well-being.

DISCLOSURE

Dr C.J. Hammond receives grant support from the National Institute on Drug Abuse, United States (NIDA; Bench to Bedside Award, R33DA056230-02W1, and K12DA000357), the American Academy of Child & Adolescent Psychiatry (AACAP), United States, the Substance Abuse and Mental Health Services Administration, United States (SAMHSA, H79 SP082126-01), the Doris Duke Charitable Foundation, United States (Grant# 2020147), the National Network of Depression Centers (NNDC), the Johns Hopkins Consortium for School-based Health Solutions, and the Johns Hopkins University School of Medicine, serves as a subject matter expert and consultant for SAMHSA, and serves on the Scientific Advisory Board for Forbes & Manhattan. Dr K. Van Eck receives grant funding from Agency for Healthcare Research and Quality, United States (AHRQ, R03HS029351), the National Institute of Child Health and Human Development, United States (NICHD, R21HD112617-01), the Centers for Disease Control and Prevention, United States (CDC, 1NU50CD300866-01-00), the Health Resources and Services Administration, United States (HRSA, 2 T16MC29832-06-00 and R42MC49146), the Office of Minority Health of the U.S. Department of Health and Human Services (CPIMP211323), and the Jessie Ball duPont Fund, United States (202103460) and provides grant review services for HRSA. Dr H. Adger is a member of the Board of Directors of the National Association for Children of Addiction (NACoA) and a Scientific Advisory board member of Smart Approaches to Marijuana (SAM).

REFERENCES

1. Casey BJ, Getz S, Galvan A. The adolescent brain. Dev Rev 2008;28(1):62–77.
2. Hammond CJ, Mayes LC, Potenza MN. Neurobiology of adolescent substance use and addictive behaviors: Prevention and treatment implications HHS public access. Adolesc Med State Art Rev 2014;25(1):15–32.
3. Bukstein OG, Horner MS. Management of the adolescent with substance use disorders and comorbid psychopathology. Child and Adolescent Psychiatric Clinics of North America 2010;19(3):609–23.
4. Manrique-Garcia E, De Leon AP, Dalman C, et al. Cannabis, psychosis, and mortality: A cohort study of 50,373 Swedish men. Am J Psychiatr 2016;173(8):790–8.
5. McGue M, Iacono WG, Krueger R. The association of early adolescent problem behavior and adult psychopathology: A multivariate behavioral genetic perspective. Behav Genet 2006;36(4):591–602.
6. Volkow ND, Baler RD, Compton WM, et al. Adverse health effects of marijuana use. N Engl J Med 2014;370(23):2219–27.
7. Tarter RE, Vanyukov M. Alcoholism: A developmental disorder. J Consult Clin Psychol 1994;62(6):1096–107.
8. Wagner FAD, Anthony JC. From first drug use to drug dependence: Developmental periods of risk for dependence upon marijuana, cocaine, and alcohol. Neuropsychopharmacology 2002;26(4):479–88. Available at: www.acnp.org/citations/Npp.

9. Hawkins JD, Catalano RF, Miller JY. Risk and protective factors for alcohol and other drug problems in adolescence and early adulthood: Implications for substance abuse prevention. Psychol Bull 1992;112(1):64–105.
10. Tao J, Ma Y, Luo C, et al. Summary of the COVID-19 epidemic and estimating the effects of emergency responses in China. Sci Rep 2021;11(1):717.
11. World Health Organization (WHO). WHO COVID-19 disease dashboard. 2024. Available at: https://data.who.int/dashboards/covid19/cases?n=c.
12. Honein MA, Christie A, Rose DA, et al. Summary of guidance for public health strategies to address high levels of community transmission of SARS-CoV-2 and related deaths, December 2020. Morb Mortal Wkly Rep 2020;69(49):1860–7.
13. Mudenda S. Letter to editor: Coronavirus Disease (COVID-19): A global health problem. International Journal of Pharmaceutics & Pharmacology 2020;4(1):1–2.
14. Bera L, Souchon M, Ladsous A, et al. Emotional and behavioral impact of the COVID-19 epidemic in adolescents. Curr Psychiatr Rep 2022;24(1):37–46.
15. Brooks SK, Webster RK, Smith LE, et al. The psychological impact of quarantine and how to reduce it: Rapid review of the evidence. Lancet 2020;395(10227): 912–20.
16. Pfefferbaum B. Children's psychological reactions to the COVID-19 pandemic. Curr Psychiatr Rep 2021;23(11):75.
17. Richter L. The effects of the COVID-19 pandemic on the risk of youth substance use. J Adolesc Health 2020;67(4):467–8.
18. Striley CW, Hoeflich CC. Converging public health crises: Substance use during the coronavirus disease 2019 pandemic. Curr Opin Psychiatr 2021;34(4):325–31.
19. Hammond CJ, Chaney A, Hendrickson B, et al. Cannabis use among U.S. adolescents in the era of marijuana legalization: A review of changing use patterns, comorbidity, and health correlates. Int Rev Psychiatr 2020;32(3):221–34.
20. Miech RA, Johnston LD, Patrick ME, et al. Monitoring the Future national survey results on drug use, 1975-2022: secondary school students. Institute for Social Research at the University of Michigan; 2023. p. 1–527.
21. Johnston LD, Miech RA, O'Malley PM, et al. Monitoring the Future national survey results on drug use,1975-2019: 2019 Overview key findings on adolescent drug use. Institute for Social Research at the University of Michigan; 2020. p. 1–131.
22. Benschop A, van Bakkum F, Noijen J. Changing patterns of substance use during the coronavirus pandemic: Self-reported use of tobacco, alcohol, cannabis, and other drugs. Front Psychiatr 2021;12:633551.
23. Chaffee BW, Cheng J, Couch ET, et al. Adolescents' substance use and physical activity before and during the COVID-19 pandemic. JAMA Pediatr 2021;175(7): 715–22.
24. Chaiton M, Dubray J, Kundu A, et al. Perceived impact of COVID on smoking, vaping, alcohol and cannabis use among youth and youth adults in Canada. Can J Psychiatr 2022;67(5):407–9.
25. Cho J, Bello MS, Christie NC, et al. Adolescent emotional disorder symptoms and transdiagnostic vulnerabilities as predictors of young adult substance use during the COVID-19 pandemic: mediation by substance-related coping behaviors. Cognit Behav Ther 2021;50(4):276–94.
26. Kuitunen I. Social restrictions due to COVID-19 and the incidence of intoxicated patients in pediatric emergency department. Ir J Med Sci 2022;191(3):1081–3.
27. McLeish AC, Hart JL, Walker KL. Long-term impact of the COVID-19 pandemic on use behavior and risk perceptions of college student E-cigarette users. J Am Coll Health 2023. https://doi.org/10.1080/07448481.2023.2194441.

28. Sen LT, Siste K, Hanafi E, et al. Insights Into adolescents' substance use in a low–middle-income country during the COVID-19 pandemic. Front Psychiatr 2021;12: 739698.

29. Thorisdottir IE, Agustsson G, Oskarsdottir SY, et al. Effect of the COVID-19 pandemic on adolescent mental health and substance use up to March, 2022, in Iceland: a repeated, cross-sectional, population-based study. The Lancet Child and Adolescent Health 2023;7(5):347–57.

30. Romm KF, Patterson B, Crawford ND, et al. Changes in young adult substance use during COVID-19 as a function of ACEs, depression, prior substance use and resilience. Subst Abuse 2022;43(1):212–21.

31. Pelham WE, Tapert SF, Gonzalez MR, et al. Early adolescent substance use before and during the COVID-19 pandemic: A longitudinal survey in the ABCD study cohort. J Adolesc Health 2021;69(3):390–7.

32. Dumas TM, Ellis W, Litt DM. What does adolescent substance use look like during the COVID-19 pandemic? Examining changes in frequency, social contexts, and pandemic-related predictors. J Adolesc Health 2020;67(3):354–61.

33. Gohari MR, Varatharajan T, Patte KA, et al. The intersection of internalizing symptoms and alcohol use during the COVID-19 pandemic: A prospective cohort study. Prev Med 2023;166:107381.

34. Layman HM, Thorisdottir IE, Halldorsdottir T, et al. Substance use among youth during the COVID-19 pandemic: A systematic review. Curr Psychiatr Rep 2022; 24(6):307–24.

35. Gaiha SM, Lempert LK, Halpern-Felsher B. Underage youth and young adult e-cigarette use and access before and during the coronavirus disease 2019 pandemic. JAMA Netw Open 2020;3(12):e2027572.

36. Creswell KG, Chung T, Wright AGC, et al. Personality, negative affect coping, and drinking alone: A structural equation modeling approach to examine correlates of adolescent solitary drinking. Addiction 2015;110(5):775–83.

37. Bahr SJ, Hoffmann JP, Yang X. Parental and peer influences on the risk of adolescent drug use. J Prim Prev 2005;26(6):529–51.

38. Staff J, Maggs JL. Parents allowing drinking is associated with adolescents' heavy alcohol use. Alcohol Clin Exp Res 2020;44(1):188–95.

39. Maggs JL, Cassinat JR, Kelly BC, et al. Parents who first allowed adolescents to drink alcohol in a family context during spring 2020 COVID-19 emergency shutdowns. J Adolesc Health 2021;68(4):816–8.

40. Friedman J, Godvin M, Shover CL, et al. Trends in drug overdose deaths among U.S. adolescents, January 2010 to June 2021. JAMA, J Am Med Assoc 2022; 327(14):1398–400.

41. Tanz LJ, Dinwiddie AT, Mattson CL, et al. Drug overdose deaths among persons aged 10–19 years — United States, July 2019–December 2021. Morb Mortal Wkly Rep 2019;71(50):1576–82. Available at: https://www.dea.gov/sites/default/files/2021-02/DIR-008-21%202020%20.

42. Hinckley JH, Hammond CJ, Yule A. Fentanyl and the opioid epidemic: Practical guidance for child and adolescent psychiatry clinicians (Clinical Perspectives 72). J Am Acad Child Adolesc Psychiatry 2023;62(10):S104–5.

43. Comer SD, Cahill CM. Fentanyl: Receptor pharmacology, abuse potential, and implications for treatment. Neurosci Biobehav Rev 2019;106:49–57.

44. Center for Disease Control and Prevention (CDC). Overdose death rates increased significantly for Black, American Indian/Alaska Native people in 2020. 2022. Available at: https://www.cdc.gov/media/releases/2022/s0719-overdose-rates-vs.html.

45. United States Drug Enforcement Administration (DEA). One pill can kill campaign. 2024. Available at: https://www.dea.gov/onepill.
46. Sawyer SM, Azzopardi PS, Wickremarathne D, et al. The age of adolescence. Lancet Child and Adolescent Health 2018;2(3):223–8.
47. World Health Organization (WHO). Adolescent and young adult health fact sheet. 2021. Available at: https://Www.Who.Int/News-Room/Fact-Sheets/Detail/Adolescent-Mentalhealth.
48. Degenhardt L, Stockings E, Patton G, et al. The increasing global health priority of substance use in young people. Lancet Psychiatr 2016;3(3):251–64.
49. Cioffredi LA, Kamon J, Turner W. Effects of depression, anxiety and screen use on adolescent substance use. Preventive Medicine Reports 2021;22:101362.
50. Zapolski TCB, Clifton RL, Banks DE, et al. Family and peer influences on substance attitudes and use among juvenile justice-involved youth. J Child Fam Stud 2019;28(2):447–56.
51. Pichel R, Feijóo S, Isorna M, et al. Analysis of the relationship between school bullying, cyberbullying, and substance use. Child Youth Serv Rev 2022;134:106369.
52. Squeglia LM, Jacobus J, Tapert SF. The Influence of substance use on adolescent brain development. Clin EEG Neurosci 2009;40(1):31–8.
53. Gray KM, Squeglia LM. Research review: What have we learned about adolescent substance use? J Child Psychol Psychiatry Allied Discip 2018;59(6):618–27.
54. Crews F, He J, Hodge C. Adolescent cortical development: A critical period of vulnerability for addiction. Pharmacol Biochem Behav 2007;86(2):189–99.
55. Crews FT, Boettiger CA. Impulsivity, frontal lobes and risk for addiction. Pharmacol Biochem Behav 2009;93(3):237–47.
56. Schulte MT, Hser Y-I. Substance use and associated health conditions throughout the lifespan. Public Health Rev 2014;35(2).
57. Brennan N, Beames JR, Kos A, et al. Psychological distress in young people in Australia fifth biennial youth mental health report: 2021-2020. Australia: Sydney, NSW: Mission; 2021. p. 1–114.
58. Bugbee BA, Beck KH, Fryer CS, et al. Substance use, academic performance, and academic engagement among high school seniors. J Sch Health 2019;89(2):145–56.
59. Rioux C, Castellanos-Ryan N, Parent S, et al. Age of cannabis use onset and adult drug abuse symptoms: A prospective study of common risk factors and indirect effects. Can J Psychiatr 2018;63(7):457–64.
60. Lubman DI, Cheetham A, Jorm AF, et al. Australian adolescents' beliefs and help-seeking intentions towards peers experiencing symptoms of depression and alcohol misuse. BMC Publ Health 2017;17(1). https://doi.org/10.1186/s12889-017-4655-3.
61. Ellonen N, Pitkänen J, Miller BL, et al. Does early drug use-related police contact predict premature mortality and morbidity: A population register-based study. Drug Alcohol Rev 2022;41(2):449–56.
62. Chaiton M, Musani I, Pullman M, et al. Access to mental health and substance use resources for 2slgbtq+ youth during the covid-19 pandemic. Int J Environ Res Publ Health 2021;18(21). https://doi.org/10.3390/ijerph182111315.
63. Akré ER, Anderson A, Stojanovski K, et al. Depression, anxiety, and alcohol use among LGBTQ+ people during the COVID-19 pandemic. Am J Publ Health 2021;111:1610–9.

64. Gould E, Kassa M. Young workers hit hard by the COVID-19 economy workers ages 16-24 face high unemployment and an uncertain future. Washington, DC: Economic Policy Institute; 2020. p. 1–23.

65. Organization for Economic Cooperation and Development. OECD policy responses to coronavirus (COVID-19): Supporting young people's mental health through the COVID-19 crisis. 2021. Available at: https://www.oecd.org/coronavirus/policy-responses/supporting-young-people-s-mental-health-through-the-covid-19-crisis-84e143e5/.

66. Koelen JA, Mansueto AC, Finnemann A, et al. COVID-19 and mental health among at-risk university students: A prospective study into risk and protective factors. Int J Methods Psychiatr Res 2022;31(1). https://doi.org/10.1002/mpr.1901.

67. Villanti AC, LePine SE, Peasley-Miklus C, et al. COVID-related distress, mental health, and substance use in adolescents and young adults. Child Adolesc Ment Health 2022;27(2):138–45.

68. Ghelbash Z, Alavi M, West S, et al. A Post-Pandemic Reset: Reversing the COVID-19 Increase in Substance Use by Adolescents and Young Adults. Issues Ment Health Nurs 2023;44(6):576–9. Taylor and Francis Ltd.

69. Nawi AM, Ismail R, Ibrahim F, et al. Risk and protective factors of drug abuse among adolescents: a systematic review. BMC Publ Health 2021;21(1):2088.

70. Diestelkamp S, Arnaud N, Sack PM, et al. Brief motivational intervention for adolescents treated in emergency departments for acute alcohol intoxication - a randomized-controlled trial. BMC Emerg Med 2014;14(1):13.

71. Winters KC, Botzet AM, Stinchfield R, et al. Adolescent substance abuse treatment: A review of evidence-based research. In: Leukefeld C, Gullotta T, editors. Adolescent substance Abuse: issues in Children's and families' lives. Springer; 2018. p. 141–71.

72. Byrnes HF, Miller BA, Grube JW, et al. Prevention of alcohol use in older teens: A randomized trial of an online family prevention program. Psychol Addict Behav 2019;33(1):1–14.

73. Horigian VE, Feaster DJ, Robbins MS, et al. A cross-sectional assessment of the long term effects of brief strategic family therapy for adolescent substance use. Am J Addict 2015;24(7):637–45.

74. Teesson M, Newton NC, Slade T, et al. Combined prevention for substance use, depression, and anxiety in adolescence: a cluster-randomised controlled trial of a digital online intervention. The Lancet Digital Health 2020;2(2):e74–84.

75. Mason M, Light J, Campbell L, et al. Peer network counseling with urban adolescents: A randomized controlled trial with moderate substance users. J Subst Abuse Treat 2015;58:16–24.

76. Substance Abuse and Mental Health Services Administration. Opioid treatment program (OTP) guidance. 2020. Available at: https://Www.Samhsa.Gov/Sites/Default/Files/Otp-Guidance-20200316.Pdf.

77. Alinsky RH, Zima BT, Rodean J, et al. Receipt of Addiction Treatment after Opioid Overdose among Medicaid-Enrolled Adolescents and Young Adults. JAMA Pediatr 2020;174(3). https://doi.org/10.1001/jamapediatrics.2019.5183.

78. American Academy of Pediatrics Committee on Substance Use And Prevention. Medication-assisted treatment of adolescents with opioid use disorders. Pediatrics 2016;138(3):e20161893.

79. Hadland SH, Aalsma MC, Akgül S, et al. Medication for adolescents and young adults with opioid use disorder. J Adolesc Health 2021;68(3):632–6.

80. Hadland SE, Yule AM, Levy SJ, et al. Evidence-based treatment of young adults with substance use disorders. Pediatrics 2021;147(2):S204–14.

81. Hammond CJ. The Role of Pharmacotherapy in the Treatment of Adolescent Substance Use Disorders. Child and Adolescent Psychiatric Clinics of North America 2016;25(4):685–711.
82. Substance Abuse and Mental Health Services Administration. Key substance use and mental health indicators in the United States: results from the 2019 national survey on drug use and health (HHS publication No. PEP20-07-01-001, NSDUH series H-55). Center for Behavioral Health Statistics and Quality, Substance Abuse and Mental Health Services Administration; 2020. Available at: https://www.samhsa.gov/data/.
83. Substance Abuse and Mental Health Services Administration. SAMHSA extends the methadone take-home flexibility for one year while working toward a permanent solution. 2021. Available at: https://Www.Samhsa.Gov/Newsroom/Press-announcements/202111181000.
84. Drug Enforcement Administration. Letter regarding doorstep delivery. 2020. Available at: https://Www.Deadiversion.Usdoj.Gov/GDP/(DEA-DC015)%20SAMHSA%20Exemption%20NTP%20Deliveries%20(CoronaVirus).Pdf.
85. Drug Enforcement Administration. Letter regarding unregistered off-site locations for methadone. 2020. Available at: https://Www.Deadiversion.Usdoj.Gov/GDP/(DEA-DC025)(DEA078)_Off-Site_OTP_delivery_method_(Final)+_esign.Pdf.
86. Drug Enforcement Administration. Letter regarding unregistered off-site locations for buprenorphine. 2020. Available at: https://Www.Deadiversion.Usdoj.Gov/GDP/(DEA-DC030)(DEA087)_off_site_otp_delivery_buprenorphine_(Esign).Pdf.
87. National Center for Drug Abuse Statistics. Drug use among youth: Facts & statistics. 2023. Available at: https://Drugabusestatistics.Org/Teen-Drug-Use/.
88. U.S. Department of Health and Human Services. Practice guidelines for the administration of Buprenorphine for treating Opioid Use Disorder; 86 FR 22439. Federal Register. 2021. Available at: https://Www.Federalregister.Gov/Documents/2021/04/28/2021- 08961/Practice-Guidelines-for-the-Administration-of-Buprenorphine-for-Treating-Opioid-Usedisorder.
89. Drug Enforcement Administration. Registration requirements for narcotic treatment programs with mobile components; 86 FR 33861. Federal Register. 2021. Available at: Https://Www.Federalregister.Gov/Documents/2021/06/28/2021-13519/Registration-Requirementsfor-Narcotic-Treatment-Programs-with-Mobile-Components.
90. Drug Enforcement Administration. How to Prescribe Controlled Substances to Patients During the COVID-19 Public Health Emergency. 2020. Available at: https://Www.Deadiversion.Usdoj.Gov/GDP/(DEA-DC023)(DEA075)Decision_Tree_(Final)_33120_2007.Pdf.
91. Drug Enforcement Administration. Letter regarding prescribing and dispensing of buprenorphine via telemedicine. 2020. Available at: https://Www.Deadiversion.Usdoj.Gov/GDP/(DEA-DC022)(DEA068)%20DEA%20SAMHSA%20buprenorphine%20telemedicine%20%20(Final)%20+Esign.Pdf.
92. Centers for Medicare & Medicaid Services. Medicare and medicaid programs: Policy and regulatory revisions in response to the COVID-19 public health emergency; 85 FR 19230. Federal Register. 2020. Available at: https://Www.Federalregister.Gov/Documents/2020/04/06/2020-06990/Medicare-and-Medicaidprograms-Policy-and-Regulatory-Revisions-in-Response-to-the-Covid-19-Public.
93. Substance Abuse and Mental Health Services Administration. Become a Buprenorphine waivered practitioner. 2022. Available at: https://Www.Samhsa.Gov/Medicationassisted-Treatment/Become-Buprenorphine-Waivered-Practitioner.

Addressing Post-Pandemic Adolescent Health in Schools

Neerav Desai, MD*, Sarah Holliday, AGPCNP-BC, WHNP-BC,
Debra Braun-Courville, MD

KEYWORDS

- Adolescent and young adult (AYA) Education • Post-pandemic education
- Digital inequality in education • Education outcomes during the pandemic

KEY POINTS

- School closures and re-opening of schools caused learning deficiencies for adolescent and young adult (AYA) across the world.
- Digital inequality affected marginalized AYA disproportionately.
- The social benefit of in-person school was reinforced by the pandemic.
- School-based health care delivery is a vital avenue to improve health care outcomes for AYA in the future.

INTRODUCTION

In May 2023, the World Health Organization and United States declared the coronavirus disease 2019 (COVID-19) public health emergency over. However, the direct and indirect consequences of the pandemic may be long-lasting, particularly in academic achievement for adolescents and young adults (AYA) aged 12 to 22. AYA are generally healthy and a large majority of COVID-19 infections in this population are associated with mild to moderate symptoms and low mortality. Yet the COVID-19 pandemic goes beyond medical risks and symptoms. We now understand that educational attainment, family dynamics, social interactions, provision of medical services, and mental health outcomes have all been negatively impacted. This may be even more pronounced for AYA who have nascent and developing coping skills. More than 1.5 billion students around the world were subject to lockdowns and school closures. The rapid transition to online instruction exacerbated existing digital inequalities, further compounding the impacts of COVID-19. Post-pandemic re-opening of schools was

Division of Adolescent and Young Adult Health, Department of Pediatrics, Vanderbilt University Medical Center, 719 Thompson Lane Suite 36300, Nashville, TN 37204, USA
* Corresponding author.
E-mail address: Neerav.desai@vumc.org

Pediatr Clin N Am 71 (2024) 671–682
https://doi.org/10.1016/j.pcl.2024.05.001   **pediatric.theclinics.com**
0031-3955/24/© 2024 Elsevier Inc. All rights reserved.

extremely heterogeneous, inconsistent, and often vacillating, all of which have placed unexpected stress on AYA. The post-pandemic world in school-aged education is an emerging field, and the long-term impacts on overall health and well-being for AYA will take years to uncover. This article describes the impact of school closures and re-openings on educational outcomes, social outcomes, and school-based health delivery for AYA.

DEFINITIONS

AYA, Adolescents and young adults, refers to those aged 12 to 22 unless otherwise stated.

SBHC, School-based health clinics.

COVID-19, Infection caused by SARS-CoV-2 virus.

IEP, Individualized Education Plan, Written educational plan to ensure that a student with a disability receives specialized education services.

504 Plan, A plan to ensure a student with a disability receives educational accommodations that will ensure academic success.

WHAT HAPPENED TO EDUCATIONAL OUTCOMES FOR ADOLESCENTS AND YOUNG ADULTS DURING THE PANDEMIC AND REINTEGRATION?

School closures interrupt the educational process and result in learning deficiencies.[1,2] In March of 2020, schools throughout the world closed to reduce the spread of COVID-19. Researchers were concerned about possible educational and psychosocial effects of these school closures. Much of the pre-pandemic educational outcome data on school closures have been extrapolated from research during school holidays or natural disasters that have impaired traditional in-person learning opportunities (Hurricane Katrina in the United States, Ebola outbreak in Sierra Leone and Guinea, and the Pakistani earthquake). Previous authors have defined a learning deficit as "both a delay in expected learning progress, as well as a loss of skills and knowledge already gained.[3]" A worldwide meta-analysis in 2023 found a substantial slowing of the learning progress during the pandemic.[3] Multiple studies show overall lower achievement in reading and math scores (as evidenced by standardized test scores) compared to pre-pandemic levels.[2,4] Unfortunately, these learning deficits were not reversed, even when in-person instruction resumed. Estimates vary, but analyses suggest that students lost out on anywhere from 10% to 30% of an academic school year due to school shutdowns.[3,5,6] Most of this learning deficit occurred early in the pandemic as school systems adapted to remote learning. Many school systems transitioned to online instruction during the pandemic to reach students and provide some structured education. However, most pre-pandemic studies have found that online learning is not equivalent to in-person instruction, independent of the quality of the program.[5]

Remote learning during the COVID-19 pandemic emphasized our dependence on technology, further amplifying the problems of digital inequality. Katz and others use the term digital inequality over the term digital divide.[8] The former implies a continuum of issues with digital learning instead of a dichotomous state implied by the word "digital divide".[8] First level digital inequality refers to unequal access to digital devices and consistent high-speed internet.[8] Connectivity issues affected rural students, and black, indigenous and other students of color disproportionally (**Table 1**).[5,7] In 2021, more than 40% of working-class families in the United States did not own a laptop or desktop computer; similar percentages did not have broadband internet connectivity.[9] Second level digital inequality refers to unequal ability by the student to utilize

Table 1	
% of K-12 students without adequate connectivity by geography and race/ethnicity	
Urban	21%
Suburban	25%
Rural	37%
White	18%
Latinx	26%
Black	30%
Native American	35%

Adapted from Chandra et al.[7]

technology in learning.[7] This often references acquired individual digital skills such as communicating via technology, optimizing devices for online learning, and trouble-shooting. Third level digital inequality refers to unequal educational outcomes in the use of technology.[8] Goudeau identifies additional digital resource limitations that may affect the learning process: printer accessibility, identification of a suitable quiet workspace, and the need for additional computers for families with multiple children.[9] Each level of digital inequality limits the learning process and overall academic student success. We have less rigorous evidence of the effect of second and third level digital inequality, but future remote learning models will have to address these inequities especially focusing on rural, racially/ethnically diverse, and other disadvantaged AYA.[8]

Remote learning during the pandemic had an adverse effect on educational out-comes for all students, but particularly AYA with autism, neurodevelopmental disor-ders, and other special needs. In 2021, parents of autistic children reported more undesirable behaviors because of pandemic school changes, including behavioral regression, increases in stimming behaviors and meltdowns, and problems with toilet-ing hygiene.[10] Other studies showed that remote learning negatively impacted coop-eration skills and self-regulation skills for children with autism.[11] Changes to established routines and schedules likely contributed to these concerns as autistic children often show a preference for sameness. AYA with attention deficit disorders (ADD/ADHD) found virtual learning to be more challenging and anxiety-provoking compared to student peers without ADHD.[12] Parents of adolescents with ADHD re-ported less confidence and more difficulties supporting their child with online learning, especially those who had a pre-existing IEP or 504 plans.[12] The sum of these experi-ences and changes affected return to in-person learning.

Recovery from learning deficit is not quick and learning outcomes are likely to be affected for years to come. Kuhfeld and Lewis posit that it "will take the average elementary school student at least 3 years to fully recover. For older students, it will take far longer. Notably, in most cases these recovery timelines extend past spending deadlines for federal recovery funds, and for some students, full recovery would not be attainable before the end of high school.[13]" Older students (7th and 8th graders) were found to have larger drops in math and reading achievement scores compared to elementary students. The authors theorize that is due to the fact that 7th and 8th graders learn more information during school so they lost more ground when schools were closed.[13] Kuhfeld and colleagues found that even in the spring 2021, nearly a full year after the start of the pandemic, academic achievement in grades 3 through 8 was still behind pre-pandemic standardized testing averages.[2] There was some evidence of academic recovery, albeit not uniform. Students who were able to catch up were generally among the more traditionally high-performing students, leading to greater variability and disparity in the classroom.[2] This heterogeneity has implications for teachers: the need to support students who are further behind and simultaneously those who are more academically on track. Academic recovery from COVID-19 learning loss is likely to be a slow process, requiring intervention on multiple levels.

HOW DO WE IMPROVE EDUCATIONAL OUTCOMES MOVING FORWARD?

The educational impacts of school closures may last for years. Learning deficits will not be completely reversed simply by returning to the classroom. The American Academy of Pediatrics and other national health organizations provided some guidance to promote in-person learning and successful educational outcomes.[14] Implementation of evidenced-based strategies to help with the post-COVID transition back to school may mitigate some of the learning loss. These strategies include: (1) early warning signals to identify students at risk who are falling behind and at-risk for dropping out, such as attendance or behavioral monitoring and course completion; (2) tutoring that is in alignment with classroom instruction; (3) improving academic performance with extended learning opportunities; (4) instructional learning programs after school and during summer or school breaks; and (5) implementation of math and reading programs.[15] Given the heterogeneity of learning experiences during the pandemic, post-pandemic academic recovery will require a multi-pronged and non-universal approach.

Guryan suggested that individualized, intensive, in-school tutoring may be one of the more effective ways to bridge the COVID-19 learning gap.[16] These authors found that 9th and 10th grade students who participated in high-impact tutoring (i.e., personalized instruction with an engaged adult outside of the normal classroom) were able to increase their standardized math test scores post-pandemic as well as demonstrate improved grades in both math and non-math courses.[16] High-impact tutoring may be an effective strategy to mitigate some of the COVID-specific learning loss. Other evidence-based interventions such as summer school, eliminating non-essential instruction, focusing on a core curriculum, and mentoring have also been identified as catch-up learning methods.[5]

WHAT WAS THE SOCIAL IMPACT OF THE PANDEMIC AND REINTEGRATION INTO SCHOOLS FOR ADOLESCENTS AND YOUNG ADULTS?

A large part of normal AYA social development is centered on school and extracurricular activities. Schools are a safe place for AYA to hone social and emotional skills, build support networks, get consistent meals, engage in physical activity, and often receive medical and therapeutic services. School connectedness refers to a student's ability to trust that "adults and peers in their school care about them, their safety, and their success".[17] Students who felt connected to and supported by their schools during the pandemic had lower prevalence of poor mental health.[18] High school students who did not feel connected to their school reported higher percentage of feelings of sadness, hopelessness, and suicidal ideation.[18] COVID-19 challenged the school system's ability to care for all youth with the loss of social protective functions. Social protective factors include in-school teacher/coach mentoring, vocational training, and other college and career counseling. AYA were deeply affected by the loss of extracurricular activities such as proms, club meetings, graduations, homecomings, sporting events, and other social bonding experiences. The loss or modification of school graduations caused a serious sense of angst amongst AYA due to the competing interests of public safety and need for social validation of their efforts.[19]

Facial coverings in schools directly impacted social experiences for AYA. Although facial coverings reduce airborne transmission of the COVID-19, face masks may also reduce the ability to communicate, interpret emotional signaling, and overall interpret facial expressions between teachers and students.[20] Mask-wearing also increases the risk of misunderstanding between individuals due to limitations in emotional recognition. This unfairly affects AYA with language and communication difficulties. For example, deaf and hearing-impaired individuals who rely on lip reading may be at a greater disadvantage when the lower half of the face is covered.[21] These social impacts of masked learning may impair bonding between classmates and teachers, and in future pandemics risks and benefits of masking in schools should be discussed transparently and openly.

AYA with social anxiety disorder and their families faced special challenges with re-opening of schools. Treatment for anxiety disorders typically involves some level of exposure to feared situations, and for AYA with social anxiety, school serves as a consistent exposure setting.[22] During the height of the COVID-19 pandemic, physical distancing and social isolation were praised, and as a result those AYA with social anxiety received positive reinforcement from actions that would typically be discouraged.[23] Avoidance of difficult situations tends to beget further avoidance, and as students entered back into schools, AYA with social anxiety have experienced acute destabilization.[23] Clinicians should be vigilant in following up with AYA that reported improved anxiety during school closures, and advocate for return to in-person schooling whenever possible, despite possible hesitancies from patients and parents who seek to continue avoidance.[23,24]

Another group that faced challenges with school closings and re-openings are those AYA that are racially diverse. Individuals in these groups experience both microaggressions and discrimination daily, and during periods of remote learning they may have felt more shielded from these daily insults.[25] For example, Asian American students reported higher levels of discontent and lower levels of belonging after school re-opening, citing racial insults and being intentionally coughed at.[26] Other studies highlight that Asian, black, and multiracial students perceived the highest rates of racism in the post-pandemic school environment and that this was correlated to worse mental health.[27] AYA became increasingly aware and vocal about racial injustices such as the "Black Lives Matter" movement during the COVID-19 pandemic and this impacted their psychological health causing "(a) anger and frustration and (b) disconnect and hopelessness".[28] This lack of belonging and connectedness can negatively impact academic performance, which can perpetuate the distress racially diverse students experience upon returning to traditional school settings.[2,25]

Sexual and gender diverse AYA experienced negative repercussions from the COVID-19 pandemic school closures and re-openings. There is ample evidence that social and structural inequality for lesbian, gay, bisexual, transgender, and questioning (LGBTQ) AYA was exacerbated during the pandemic.[29] School aged LGBTQ individuals were more likely to be living in poverty and less likely to be insured. They often depend on school-based services such as counseling and nutrition programs.[30] Connectedness is important for LGBTQ adolescents and social isolation reduced access to safe affirming communities such as gender and sexual alliances and supportive school personnel.[31] As LGBTQ youth re-enter school, we will need to support them through increased accessibility to on-line counseling, leveraging social media for connectedness, and re-emphasizing the importance of affirming social spaces for their continued well-being.[29]

During the COVID-19 pandemic, AYA utilized the Internet and social media in even greater rates than previously.[25] Social interactions are generally seen as satisfying when they contain rich sensory information and opportunity for bodily feedback.[32] So-cial media-based interactions and applications provide the first component of rich sensory information, but they miss the critical opportunity for face-to-face interac-tions, providing positive, but fleeting, emotional stimulation. An increase in social me-dia usage during lockdowns led students to immerse themselves more and more into the online world, which can make it harder to perceive the emotional value of in-person social interactions, unintentionally perpetuating the social isolation experienced at the height of the COVID-19 pandemic.[32,33]

HOW DO WE GUIDE SCHOOLS FOR ADOLESCENTS AND YOUNG ADULT'S SOCIAL NEEDS IN THE FUTURE?

As students begin to re-enter the post-pandemic learning environment, community health experts posit that schools should focus on providing as much in-person inter-action as possible.[14] This means tailoring education methods to include more discussion-based learning, group projects, and interactive pedagogical methods, despite the seeming convenience of virtual classrooms and traditional lecture-based methods.[34] Young Minds UK advocates that social well-being be made a pri-ority at schools, specifically avoiding the impulse to focus on simply "catching up" academically.[35] Research has long found that social interactions with one's peer group enhances positive social behaviors in AYA, including cooperation and empathy, and reduces problem behaviors in the classroom, which can make the task of aca-demic restoration that much easier.[25,36] Examples of these social opportunities could include extracurricular activities such as prom, homecoming, sporting events, club participation, as well as informal gatherings such as spirit days, school picnics, and opportunities to connect with faculty and staff outside of the classroom or administra-tive setting. Safe return to school-sponsored sports participation can also facilitate so-cial interactions and skills building.[14]

SCHOOL-BASED HEALTH DELIVERY CHANGES DURING THE PANDEMIC AND REINTEGRATION INTO SCHOOL

School-based health clinics (SBHC) can be a vital resource for delivery of health care and health promotion. In many cases SBHC serve as a medical home for youth and present an avenue for comprehensive care which they would not have otherwise particularly in urban and rural settings. Widespread school lockdowns also forced SBHC closures.[37] The pandemic impacted school-based health delivery of primary care services for AYA (**Table 2**). This includes services that many AYA cannot access at a primary care office due to constraints in geography, time, transportation, and other structural barriers. Disruptions in service delivery of SBHC can affect the overall health of AYA. A delay in some of the primary care services offered, such as hearing and vision screening, may have a direct impact on academic performance. Other ser-vices, such as influenza and COVID vaccinations, can prevent missed time from school or learning. In one study, dental screenings showed the largest decline asso-ciated with the pandemic.[38]

More than half of SBHC provide behavioral health services.[39] Virginia school nurses surveyed in 2022 reported access to mental health care as a top priority for AYA stu-dents during the pandemic, particularly with return to in-person schooling.[38] At the same time this developing need was emerging, SBHC were less likely to provide behavioral health services to students in the 2020 to 2021 school year compared to pre-pandemic service delivery.[38] Service provision disruption, inadequate staffing, and competing provider responsibilities likely contributed to diminished resources.

Table 2	
School-based health delivery disruptions during the pandemic	
Primary Care	Immunizations
	Vision and Hearing Screening
	Dental Screening
Episodic Care	Triaging
	Asthma Management
	Allergic Reactions
	Seizure Management
	Sports Injuries
Mental Health	School-Based Counseling
	Acute mental health or substance crisis management/ de-escalation
Services for AYA with special needs	Speech and Language therapy
	Occupational Therapy
	Physical Therapy
	Applied Behavioral Analysis

Health care delivery for AYA with autism spectrum, neurodevelopmental disorders, and other special needs was heavily impacted by school closures. In-school special education services coordinated by SBHC such as occupational, physical, speech, and applied behavioral analysis were likely disrupted, further leading to negative consequences for AYA with special needs.[40] This disruption of services affected low-income families disproportionately.[40] Virtual learning and support services for autistic, neurodivergent, and other special needs AYA may have been less effective and not adequate to meet student needs due to communication barriers.[10]

Perhaps the biggest impact of the pandemic on school-based health delivery has been on the workforce that delivers the care, namely school nurses. School nurses took on additional job responsibilities during the pandemic: devising and implementing mitigation strategies to reduce school transmission; contacting students and guardians about isolation and quarantine guidelines; and providing care for individuals (students, staff, and teachers) with confirmed or suspected COVID-19 infections.[41] School nurses often led implementation of mitigation strategies such as physical distancing, mask wearing, hand hygiene practices, and ventilation and air purification programs.[42] This pulled them away from other vital needs such as primary care prevention, sexual health education, injury and violence prevention, and mental health triaging.[41] School nurses faced additional personal challenges during the pandemic such as, increased rates of mental health conditions like depression, anxiety, post-traumatic stress disorder, and suicidal ideation compared to the general United States population.[43] The monumental need in primary care and mental health care services for AYA after the pandemic, may further stress the school nurse workforce in the future.

THE FUTURE OF SCHOOL-BASED HEALTH DELIVERY

In the future, SBHC will need to adapt to the highly variable post-pandemic school conditions. SBHC can help AYA catch-up on preventive health care and maintenance including vaccinations, dental care, vision screens, hearing assessments, and sports-related pre-participation examinations.[37] Restoration and provision of mental health care services will be paramount. The American Academy of Pediatrics recently called for increased implementation and provision of sustainable mental health services in the school-based health setting to address this mismatch of increased need and reduced availability of mental health support.[44] School health systems may consider the following adaptations upon re-opening as suggested by Kranz and the AAP.[14,38,44]:

1. Acknowledge that schools provide more than just education for students. They should also prioritize AYA overall well-being.
2. Engage with community-based organizations and health departments to identify and safely meet the overall health needs of school children and adolescents.
3. Partner with SBHC to create natural disaster and/or future pandemic preparedness plans to safeguard the physical and mental health of school-aged children.
4. Collaborate with local vaccine clinics to provide equitable distribution of vaccines, including COVID-19 vaccination.
5. Advocate for staff and family support for SBHC.
6. Recognize and address the mental health needs of students. Consider federal and state funding options to develop community partnerships and/or hiring of in-school social workers and behavioral health specialists in SBHC.
7. SBHC will need to adopt telehealth modalities for delivering some types of care including counseling services.[37]
8. Consider school-based problem-solving therapy with a school counselor as an initial step for mental health concerns with the ability to escalate care as needed.[45,46]

These adaptations will likely be associated with a steep learning curve to meet the needs of AYA and achieve sustainability. Key issues that will affect the future of SBHC health care delivery include confidentiality, reimbursement, and evidence of financial and health care outcome benefits.[37] See **Table 3**.

Table 3
Emerging school-based health clinic (SBHC) telehealth delivery models[37]

Telehealth Model	SBHC Telehealth Innovations
Launching telehealth	• Providing primary care telemedicine • Providing telebehavioral health
Expanding telehealth	• Expansion of services to include telemedicine, telebehavioral health, or teledentistry • Expanding clientele served outside of the school • Collaboration with specialty clinics (eg, obesity specialty) • Increase in telehealth visits (eg, 15 visits/month to 857 visits/month)
Altering telehealth	• Telehealth COVID-19 screening before in-person care • Telehealth screening visits before physical examinations • Existing patients moved from in-person to telehealth visits • Lower threshold for patients referrals to in-person care • More frequent follow-up with patients (eg, "touchpoints") • Mail-home STI kits with telehealth follow-up • Telehealth "senior transition" visits to adult care • Primary care providers doing mental health visits • Telehealth reproductive health counseling and prescriptions • Changing SBHC hours into the evening

Note: COVID-19, coronavirus disease 2019, STI, sexually transmitted infections.

SUMMARY

In summary, pandemic school closures and re-opening of schools universally represented a challenge to AYA, their families, and school systems. We have strong evidence of long-lasting learning deficits which will take years to address. Learning deficiencies were compounded by digital inequalities which affected marginalized AYA disproportionately. Recovery from the learning deficits will take concerted effort and sustained funding. We have strong evidence of the social benefits of in-person school learning and the social fabric of schools will need to be addressed in the re-opening of schools. We recognize that SBHC have a vital role in restoring the physical and mental tolls of the pandemic for AYA in the future. As such, SBHC will need to be supported by families, communities, and government funding.

CLINICS CARE POINTS

- Pediatric and adolescent primary care providers will need to be aware of the learning deficiencies that were exacerbated by the pandemic. Pediatric and adolescent primary care providers can advocate for evidence-based ways of improving academic outcomes such as high impact individualized tutoring, extended learning programs, and mentoring programs for vocational goals.

- Pediatric and adolescent primary care providers can advocate for the importance of social connectedness that comes from in-person schooling.

- Pediatric and adolescent primary care providers can support and communicate with school-based health clinics to improve the physical and mental health of AYA.

DISCLOSURE

The authors of this article declare that they have no commercial interests, financial interests, or funding sources to disclose as it relates to this topic and this article.

REFERENCES

1. Marcotte D, Hemelt SW. Unscheduled School Closings and Student Performance. Education Finance and Policy 2008;3(3):316–38.
2. Kuhfeld M, Soland J, Lewis K, et al. The COVID-19 School Year: Learning and Recovery Across 2020-2021. AERA Open 2022;8. 23328584221099306.
3. Betthauser BA, Bach-Mortensen AM, Engzell P. A systematic review and meta-analysis of the evidence on learning during the COVID-19 pandemic. Nat Hum Behav 2023;7(3):375–85.
4. Rose S, Badr K, Fletcher L, et al. Impact of School Closures and subsequent support strategies on attainment and socio-emotional wellbeing in Key Stage 1. Research Report, Education Endowment Foundation, 2021. Available at: https://files.eric.ed.gov/fulltext/ED620409.pdf. Accessed August 3, 2023.
5. Dorn E, Hancock B, Sarakatsannis J, Viruleg E. COVID-19 and student learning in the United States: the hurt could last a lifetime. Report, McKinsey & Company, 2020. Available at: https://www.mckinsey.com/industries/education/our-insights/covid-19-and-student-learning-in-the-united-states-the-hurt-could-last-a-lifetime. Accessed August 24, 2023.
6. Engzell P, Frey A, Verhagen MD. Learning loss due to school closures during the COVID-19 pandemic. Proc Natl Acad Sci U S A 2021;118(17).

7. Chandra S,CA, Day L, Liu J, et al. Closing the K-12 digital Divide in the age of distance learning. Boston Consulting Group; 2020.

8. Katz VS, Jordan AB, Ognyanova K. Digital inequality, faculty communication, and remote learning experiences during the COVID-19 pandemic: A survey of U.S. undergraduates. PLoS One 2021;16(2):e0246641.

9. Goudeau S, Sanrey C, Stanczak A, et al. Why lockdown and distance learning during the COVID-19 pandemic are likely to increase the social class achievement gap. Nat Hum Behav 2021;5(10):1273–81.

10. Genova HM, Arora A, Boticello AL. Effects of School Closures Resulting from COVID-19 in Autistic and Neurotypical Children. Frontiers In Education 2021;6.

11. Morris PO, Hope E, Foulsham T, et al. Parent-reported social-communication changes in children diagnosed with autism spectrum disorder during the COVID-19 pandemic in the UK. Int J Dev Disabil 2023;69(2):211–25.

12. Becker SP, Breaux R, Cusick CN, et al. Remote Learning During COVID-19: Examining School Practices, Service Continuation, and Difficulties for Adolescents With and Without Attention-Deficit/Hyperactivity Disorder. J Adolesc Health 2020;67(6):769–77.

13. Kuhfeld M, Lewis K. Student Achievment in 2021-22: Case for hope and continued urgency, Northwest Evaluation Association, Editor, 2022. Available at: https://www.nwea.org/uploads/2022/07/Student-Achievement-in-2021-22-Cause-for-hope-and-concern.researchbrief-1.pdf. Accessed September 12, 2023.

14. COVID-19 Guidance for Safe Schools and Promotion of In-Person Learning. Publisher American Academy of Pediatrics, 2022. Available at: https://www.aap.org/en/pages/2019-novel-coronavirus-covid-19-infections/clinical-guidance/covid-19-planning-considerations-return-to-in-person-education-in-schools/?_ga=2.13421 1278.1968804256.1717426788-372129869.1717426521. Accessed August 1, 2023.

15. Kwakye I, Kibort-Crocker E. Facing learning disruption: Examining the effects of the COVID-19 pandemic on K-12 students, Washington Student Achievement Council, Editor, 2021. Available at: https://wsac.wa.gov/sites/default/files/2021-03-30-COVID-Learning-Disruption-Report.pdf. Accessed September 12, 2023.

16. Guryan J, Ludwig J, Bhatt MP, et al. Not Too Late: Improving Academic Outcomes among Adolescents. Am Econ Rev 2023;113(3):738–65.

17. Krause KH, Mpofu JJ, Underwood JM, et al. The CDC's Adolescent Behaviors and Experiences Survey - Using Intersectionality and School Connectedness to Understand Health Disparities During the COVID-19 Pandemic. J Adolesc Health 2022;70(5):703–5.

18. Jones SE, Ethier KA, Hertz M, et al. Mental Health, Suicidality, and Connectedness Among High School Students During the COVID-19 Pandemic - Adolescent Behaviors and Experiences Survey, United States, January-June 2021. MMWR Suppl 2022;71(3):16–21.

19. Mueller AS, Diefendorf S, Abrutyn S, et al. Youth Mask-Wearing and Social-Distancing Behavior at In-Person High School Graduations During the COVID-19 Pandemic. J Adolesc Health 2021;68(3):464–71.

20. Spitzer M. Masked education? The benefits and burdens of wearing face masks in schools during the current Corona pandemic. Trends Neurosci Educ 2020;20:100138.

21. Schafer EC, Dunn A, Lavi A. Educational Challenges During the Pandemic for Students Who Have Hearing Loss. Lang Speech Hear Serv Sch 2021;52(3):889–98.

22. Banneyer KN, Bonin L, Price K, et al. Cognitive Behavioral Therapy for Childhood Anxiety Disorders: a Review of Recent Advances. Curr Psychiatry Rep 2018; 20(8):65.
23. Morrissette M. School Closures and Social Anxiety During the COVID-19 Pandemic. J Am Acad Child Adolesc Psychiatry 2021;60(1):6–7.
24. Loades ME, Chatburn E, Higson-Sweeney N, et al. Rapid Systematic Review: The Impact of Social Isolation and Loneliness on the Mental Health of Children and Adolescents in the Context of COVID-19. J Am Acad Child Adolesc Psychiatry 2020;59(11):1218–1239 e3.
25. Ni Y, Jia F. Promoting Positive Social Interactions: Recommendation for a Post-Pandemic School-Based Intervention for Social Anxiety. Children 2023;10(3).
26. Dong F, Hwang Y, Hodgson NA. Relationships between racial discrimination, social isolation, and mental health among international Asian graduate students during the COVID-19 pandemic. J Am Coll Health 2022;1–8.
27. Mpofu JJ, Cooper AC, Ashley C, et al. Perceived Racism and Demographic, Mental Health, and Behavioral Characteristics Among High School Students During the COVID-19 Pandemic - Adolescent Behaviors and Experiences Survey, United States, January-June 2021. MMWR Suppl 2022;71(3):22–7.
28. Yeh CJ, Stanley S, Ramirez CA, et al. Navigating the "Dual Pandemics": The Cumulative Impact of the COVID-19 Pandemic and Rise in Awareness of Racial Injustices among High School Students of Color in Urban Schools. Urban Educ 2022. 00420859221097884.
29. Salerno JP, Williams ND, Gattamorta KA. LGBTQ populations: Psychologically vulnerable communities in the COVID-19 pandemic. Psychol Trauma 2020; 12(S1):S239–42.
30. Zhang L, Finan LJ, Bersamin M, et al. Sexual Orientation-Based Depression and Suicidality Health Disparities: The Protective Role of School-Based Health Centers. J Res Adolesc 2020;30(Suppl 1):134–42.
31. Kaniuka A, Pugh KC, Jordan M, et al. Stigma and suicide risk among the LGBTQ population: Are anxiety and depression to blame and can connectedness to the LGBTQ community help? J Gay Lesb Ment Health 2019;23(2):205–20.
32. Costa RM, Patrao I, Machado M. Problematic internet use and feelings of loneliness. Int J Psychiatry Clin Pract 2019;23(2):160–2.
33. Brailovskaia J, Miragall M, Margraf J, et al. The relationship between social media use, anxiety and burden caused by coronavirus (COVID-19) in Spain. Curr Psychol 2022;41(10):7441–7.
34. Long E, Patterson S, Maxwell K, et al. COVID-19 pandemic and its impact on social relationships and health. J Epidemiol Community Health 2022;76(2):128–32.
35. The Impact of Covid-19 on young people with mental health needs, Young Minds UK, Editor. 2021. Available at: https://www.youngminds.org.uk/media/esifqn3z/youngminds-coronavirus-report-jan-2021.pdf. Accessed September 25, 2023.
36. Durlak JA, Weissberg RP, Pachan M. A meta-analysis of after-school programs that seek to promote personal and social skills in children and adolescents. Am J Community Psychol 2010;45(3–4):294–309.
37. Goddard A, Sullivan E, Fields P, et al. The future of telehealth in school-based health centers: lessons from COVID-19. J Pediatr Health Care 2021;35(3):304–9.
38. Kranz AM, Steiner ED, Mitchell JM. School-Based Health Services in Virginia and the COVID-19 Pandemic. J Sch Health 2022;92(5):436–44.
39. Anderson S, Haeder S, Caseman K, et al. When Adolescents are in School During COVID-19, Coordination Between School-Based Health Centers and Education is Key. J Adolesc Health 2020;67(6):745–6.

40. Bhat A. Analysis of the SPARK study COVID-19 parent survey: Early impact of the pandemic on access to services, child/parent mental health, and benefits of on-line services. Autism Res 2021;14(11):2454–70.
41. Barbee-Lee M, Seymour K, Hett AL, et al. School Nursing in a Pandemic: Striving for Excellence in Santa Fe Public Schools. NASN Sch Nurse 2021;36(5):276–83.
42. McLeod RS, Hopfe CJ, Bodenschatz E, et al. A multi-layered strategy for COVID-19 infection prophylaxis in schools: A review of the evidence for masks, distancing, and ventilation. Indoor Air 2022;32(10):e13142.
43. Merkle SL, Welton M, van Zyl A, et al. Symptoms of Depression, Anxiety, and Post-Traumatic Stress Disorder, and Suicidal Ideation Among School Nurses in Prekindergarten through Grade 12 Schools - United States, March 2022. J Sch Nurs 2023;39(2):114–24.
44. AAP-AACAP-CHA Declaration of a National Emergency in Child and Adolescent Mental Health Policy Statement. Available at: https://www.aap.org/en/advocacy/child-and-adolescent-healthy-mental-development/aap-aacap-cha-declaration-of-a-national-emergency-in-child-and-adolescent-mental-health/. Accessed April 2, 2024.
45. Michelson D, Malik K, Parikh R, et al. Effectiveness of a brief lay counsellor-delivered, problem-solving intervention for adolescent mental health problems in urban, low-income schools in India: a randomised controlled trial. Lancet Child Adolesc Health 2020;4(8):571–82.
46. Metz K, Lewis J, Mitchell J, et al. Problem-solving interventions and depression among adolescents and young adults: A systematic review of the effectiveness of problem-solving interventions in preventing or treating depression. PLoS One 2023;18(8):e0285949.

Social Media Use During Coronavirus Disease 2019 and the Impact on Adolescent Health

LaKeshia N. Craig, MD[a],*,
Renata Arrington-Sanders, MD, MPH, ScM[b,1]

KEYWORDS

- Social media • Adolescents • Young adults • Post-pandemic • COVID-19

KEY POINTS

- Social media usage increased during the coronavirus disease 2019 lockdown.
- Adolescents and young adults use a variety of social media platforms, and the popularity of the applications change over time.
- Social media can place adolescents at risk for mood disorder disturbances, attention problems, cyberbullying, sexual solicitation, and high-risk behaviors.
- Social media can have benefits including connectivity, networking, health information, and education.
- Post-pandemic social media use and effects are a new area of interest but trends show that usage is returning to prepandemic rates in younger adolescents.

INTRODUCTION

The coronavirus disease 2019 (COVID-19) pandemic irrevocably altered the lives of adolescents worldwide. Shelter-in-place order limited in-person interactions for many adolescents causing social interactions to take place virtually on digital formats including an assortment of social media platforms, with certain social media applications seeing a growth of active users worldwide by up to 38%.[1] Most (95%) adolescents in the United States report having smart phone access, with nearly 50% reporting being on social media "constantly."[2] In one study, adolescents aged 10 to 13 years that used social media between 2 and 6 hours per day increased from 2%

[a] Division of Adolescent Medicine, Department of Pediatrics, Medical University of South Carolina, Summey Medical Pavilion, 2250 Mall Drive, Floor 2, North Charleston, SC 29406, USA; [b] Craig-Dalsimer Division of Adolescent Medicine, Department of Pediatrics, Children's Hospital of Philadelphia, 3501 Civic Center Boulevard, Philadelphia, PA 19104, USA
[1] Present address: HUB, 14th Floor, Office# 14581.
* Corresponding author.
E-mail address: craiglak@musc.edu

Pediatr Clin N Am 71 (2024) 683–691
https://doi.org/10.1016/j.pcl.2024.05.003
0031-3955/24/© 2024 Elsevier Inc. All rights reserved, including those for text and data mining, AI training, and similar technologies.
pediatric.theclinics.com

prepandemic to 12% during the pandemic and those that used greater than 6 hours of social media per day increased from 0.5% to 2%. Whereas adolescents that used less than 1 hour of social media decreased from 92% to 72% during the pandemic.[3,4]

OVERVIEW OF SOCIAL MEDIA

Social media is defined as Web sites and applications that enable users to create and share content or to participate in social networking.[4] Common Web sites and applications include Facebook and Snapchat; recently social media has expanded to include gaming (Roblox, Roblox Corporation San Mateo, CA), fitness (MyFitnessPal, Francisco Partners San Francisco, CA), and business (LinkedIn, LinkedIn Corporation Sunnyvale, CA) applications, making it difficult to avoid social media.[5] In 2023, the top social media platforms (**Fig. 1**), according to Pew Research Center, were YouTube (Google San Bruno, CA), TikTok (ByteDance Singapore and Los Angeles, CA), Snapchat (Snap Inc. Santa Monica, CA), Instagram (Meta Platforms Inc, Menlo Park, CA), Facebook (Meta Platforms Inc., Menlo Park, CA), Discord (Discord Inc, San Francisco, CA), WhatsApp (Meta Platforms Inc, Mountain View, CA), Twitter (X) (X Corp, San Francisco, CA), Twitch (Amazon Interactive, San Francisco, CA), Reddit (Advance Publications, San Francisco, CA), and BeReal (Alexis Barreyat and Kevin Perrau).[2]

Use varies by platform type and function. In 2023, 93% of adolescents reported using YouTube, an online video-sharing and streaming platform,[6] and 16% of adolescents stated they "almost constantly" are on YouTube.[2] In 2023, 63% of adolescents reported using TikTok, a video hosting service, and 17% of adolescents stated that they "almost constantly" are on TikTok.[2] In 2018, TikTok merged with Musical.ly another short video platform[7] expanding TikTok's video capacity to include special effects and audio to enhance its content and use. Use of Instagram, a photograph and video-sharing service with location tagging,[8] was 59% among adolescents, up 7% from use in 2014 to 2015%, and 8% of adolescents stated they "almost constantly" are on Instagram.[2] Facebook is still a commonly used social media platform, but use by adolescents has dropped from 71% in 2014 to 2015 to only 33% in 2023.[2]

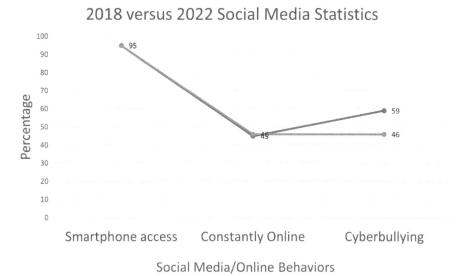

Fig. 1. Social media/online behavior.

All platforms are not solely used for social media and entertainment and have been utilized for other areas like education, training, advertisement, possibly inflating the number of users who have ever used the Web site/application for social media.

An important aspect of social media to consider is the "algorithm." The algorithm is utilized by social media platforms to push favorable content to the consumer. In other words, the algorithm learns the users likes and dislikes and feeds them content that might be interesting or well received. This can be favorable to a consumer as they can see preferred content and discover new and interesting content as well. It can also be harmful in that negative or damaging content that the algorithm deems important to the viewer is propagated.[9]

POSITIVE BENEFITS OF SOCIAL MEDIA

Social media is a tool that can promote key tasks of adolescence, including relationship building with peers, social development, and autonomy.[10] It allows for convenient ways to directly communicate with peers, and social network members, as well as share information with anyone in one's social circle.[11–13] During COVID-19, social media provided adolescents with similar interactions as in-person connections (eg, affirmative responses such as likes to behavior), video messaging platforms that provided visual support, and community discussion boards that provided a space to talk about events and cope with the pandemic.[14] According to data from the Pew Research Center, in a sample of 1316 adolescents, aged 13 to 17 years, surveyed between April and May 2022, 80% of adolescents stated that social media allows them to feel more connected with what is going on with their friends, 67% stated social media allows them to have people in their lives that can support them, and 58% stated social media allows them to feel more accepted. A small group stated that social media has improved their mental health and well-being. Only 9% stated that social media had a mostly negative impact.[15]

In a separate study of 2165 Flemish students aged between 13 and 19 years, the authors demonstrated that social media serves different coping purposes for adolescents who were anxious or lonely during the lockdown.[11] The authors sought to determine whether different social media coping strategies (active, social relations, and humor) mediated the relationship between anxiety and loneliness with happiness and found that anxious adolescents utilized social media to adapt to current situations and manage feelings of crisis, and this coping strategy had a positive relationship with feelings of happiness. Adolescents who reported being lonely, however, were more inclined to use social media as a coping strategy for loneliness, but this was not associated with feelings of happiness.[11] This study suggests that social media may have positive coping benefits, particularly for adolescents who report being anxious.

Social media also provides many adolescents with access to nontraditional forms of education. In survey of 872 undergraduate students in the United States (mean age 22 years), 44% of the students expressed that social media helped the transition to virtual learning. Students who used greater than 5 hours of social media per day reported that social media was beneficial to transitioning to virtual learning compared to those who reported less than 2 hours per day.[16] In a study examining 431 university and postgraduate students in India, 77% of male individuals and 60% of female individuals found social media helped them improve their grade during the pandemic and 33% of male individuals and 45% of female individuals noted a highly positive impact on academic performance. In contrast, only 11% of male individuals and 39% of female individuals reported a highly negative impact. Both male individuals and female individuals reported YouTube as their preferred social media platform.[17]

Social media has other health benefits. It provides access to important health information; during the COVID-19 pandemic, this included health information related how to prevent the spread of COVID-19, access to testing modalities, and information about risk from reputable sources (eg, World Health Organization and Centers for Disease Control and Prevention).[18] It is a critical tool to helping to reach hard-to-reach populations at risk for disadvantage (youth, older adults, low socioeconomic status, and rural).[19] Additionally, more research suggests that social media is an effective tool to engage adolescents in studies, disseminate information, and implement public health interventions.[20]

NEGATIVE IMPACT OF SOCIAL MEDIA

In a meta-analysis of 30 studies examining the effect of social media use on well-being, the authors found that increased time spent on social media was positively correlated with ill-being (k = 11, r = 0.171, 95% CI [0.050–0.286], P = .011, I2 = 96%), indicating that using social media platforms as related to higher psychological symptoms.[21] This relationship was augmented by age and assigned male gender. More negative effects were found in persons with greater use. The authors did highlight that the negative effects of social media were not universal—one-on-one communication, self-disclosure in the context of a mutual online friendship, and positive online feelings mitigated feelings of loneliness and stress. In single studies included in the analysis that examined ill-being, higher social media use was associated with higher levels of depression, anxiety, and lower self-esteem, especially among persons assigned female gender.[22,23] This is in-line with other study that has demonstrated that more time using social media during COVID-19 lockdown was associated with higher rates of psychological distress and depression, and this relationship was greater than periods in the pre-COVID-19 period.[24,25]

According to the National Center for Health Research, social isolation can result from increased social media use. In a study of 32 teenagers, aged 13 to 18 years, by the University of California, Los Angeles (UCLA) Brain Mapping Center, researchers used functional MRI to examine how the teenage brain would respond to likes and images in a social network like phone-sharing app. Researchers showed images on a computer screen for 12 minutes, including photographs that the teen participants submitted, with associated likes supposedly received from other participants. Higher number of likes on posted photographs was associated with increased activity in the reward center of the teenagers' brain, suggesting a positive response, whereas lower likes or negative comments could have an opposite effect.[26] Such social media responses can also contribute an adolescent's risk for cyberbullying and cybervictimization.[27]

Increased social media use during COVID-19 was also associated with increased eating disorder (ED) behavior, which was thought to be multifactorial. Initial stay at home orders early in the COVID-19 pandemic contributed to antifat fear or fear of weight gain in the setting of social isolation.[28–31] Social media simultaneously exposed adolescents to forums and virtual spaces that supported those with ED-specific behavior.[22,23] In a study examining body image and social media use during the pandemic among 2601 women aged 14 to 35 years (mean age 24 years) where 62% of participants were aged 14 to 24 years, the proportion of YouTube, Instagram, TikTok, Twitter, and Facebook use and the number of women following appearance-centered accounts increased significantly in all age groups during the pandemic. In the group with participants aged 14 to 24 years, those who followed appearance-centered Instagram accounts experienced worse body dissatisfaction and a higher drive for thinness compared to those followed other types of accounts.[32] Other data suggest that the negative impact of social media image filters continued after COVID-19, with adolescents and young adults aged 18 to 24 years using image filters having higher rates than adults of anxiety and mental health returning to in-person activities and reporting a desire change their appearance.[33]

SOCIAL MEDIA AFTER PANDEMIC

A few studies suggest that social media use among adolescents appears to be returning to pre-COVID-19 levels (**Fig. 2**). In a study of 477 Swiss adolescents (mean age 14 years), parents were asked to complete an online survey regarding their children's media time before, during, and after the pandemic. Parents noted that their adolescent's social media usage increased during the lockdown but decreased after the lockdown and has returned to near prepandemic levels in all genders. The only exception noted is that male gaming has remained higher than prepandemic levels but still lower than during the lockdown.[34] In a separate study of Turkish adolescents, adolescents were surveyed prepandemic (August 2019–February 2022) and post-pandemic (March 2022–September 2022) to determine media usage before and after the pandemic. The Smartphone Addiction Scale (SAS), the Internet Gaming Disorder Scale 9-Short Form (IGDS9-SF), and the Social Media Disorder Scale-Short Form (SMDS-SF) were filled out by the participants. The study found no significant differences of the SAS, IGDS9-SF, or SMDS-SF scores prepandemic versus post-pandemic.[35] The post-pandemic response for this study was moderate at only 40%, thus limiting the study, it does suggest that use is similar to prepandmic levels. Additional smartphone metrics suggest that both percent of adolescents with smartphone use and percent of a constantly online has remained around 95% and 45% in 2018 and 2022.[2,36] While smartphone access is not equivalent to social media use, it does demonstrate that there has not been an increase in the most convenient tool to view social media.

More data are needed to examine post-pandemic social media usage and the impact of use on adolescent behavior. Current publications predominantly representative of timeframes immediately post-COVID-19 surge. Few longitudinal studies have been conducted in the post-pandemic era to determine the causal relationship between social media use and adverse health outcomes, particularly mental health, and brain development.[37] More research is needed to distinguish the impact of social media from all screen media on mental health and other health outcomes. There is a

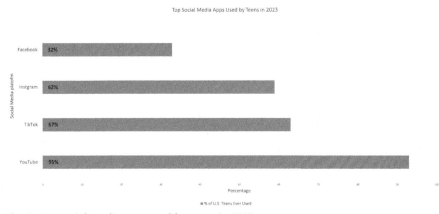

Fig. 2. Top social media apps used by teens in 2023.

lack of information around the amounts, types, and content of social media that are most harmful to adolescent development, and which may promote risk and resilience factors.

SUMMARY

The COVID-19 pandemic predisposed many adolescents to anxiety, depression, and isolation. Social media had both positive and negative benefits during the pandemic that simultaneously contributed to negative health outcomes for some and provided an outlet for coping for others. Current data suggest that adolescents may be susceptible to the negative consequences of social media usage, and supervision is critical for safe consumption. Parents, educators, and providers will need to continue to engage adolescents in an open dialog around the benefits and risks of excessive social media use and to help adolescents set boundaries to help them manage use effectively.

CLINICS CARE POINTS

Adapted from American Academy of Pediatrics social media anticipatory guidance.[5]

Physicians can provide the following anticipatory guidance for school-age children, adolescents, and caregivers:

- Encourage active engagement among parents rather than passive viewing.
  - Develop a social media contract with adolescents, reviewing limitations and use.
  - Select and coview media with their adolescents, with a focus on family and community engagement.
  - Have ongoing communication with adolescents about online citizenship (eg, treating others with respect online) and safety.
  - Discuss with adolescents the harmful impact of cyberbullying and sexting.
- Encourage families to place appropriate limits on media to mitigate negative effects and avoid displacement of healthier activities.
  - Consider using apps to limit Internet access based on content or time of day.
  - Designate media-free mealtimes (eg, dinner) and zones (eg, bedrooms).
  - Discourage media use during homework outside of what is needed to complete the assignment; consider placing devices in a central location so that parents can monitor that use is for schoolwork.
- Encourage parents to model the digital behavior they expect from their adolescents.

DISCLOSURE

The authors have nothing to disclose.

FUNDING

Dr R. Arrington-Sanders is funded by the National Institute of Health (1R01DA043089, 1R01DA059022) and receives royalties for serving as a section editor for UpToDate, Wolters Kluwer.

REFERENCES

1. Dixon SJ. Social media platforms mau growth 2021. Statista; 2023. Available at: https://www.statista.com/statistics/1219318/social-media-platforms-growth-of-mau-worldwide/. [Accessed 3 September 2023].

2. Anderson M, Faverio M, Gottfried J. Teens, social media and technology 2023. Pew Research Center: Internet, Science & Tech; 2023. Available at: https://www.pewresearch.org/internet/2023/12/11/teens-social-media-and-technology-2023/.

3. Kiss O, Nagata JM, de Zambotti M, et al. Effects of the COVID-19 pandemic on screen time and sleep in early adolescents. Health Psychol 2023;42(12): 894–903. American Psychological Association.

4. Social media - Oxford English Dictionary. Available at: www.oed.com https://www.oed.com/search/dictionary/?scope=Entries&q=social+media&tl=true.

5. Hill DL. Social Media: Anticipatory Guidance. Pediatr Rev 2020;41(3):112–9.

6. Hosch WL. YouTube. In: Encyclopedia britannica. 2019. Available at: https://www.britannica.com/topic/YouTube.

7. TikTok | App History, Videos, China, & Controversies | Britannica. Available at: https://www.britannica.com/topic/TikTok.

8. Eldrige A. Britannica Academic. academic.eb.com. Available at: https://academic.eb.com/levels/collegiate/article/Instagram/627874. [Accessed 2 October 2023].

9. Petrescu M, Krishen AS. The dilemma of social media algorithms and analytics. Journal of Marketing Analytics 2020;8(4):187–8.

10. Christie D, Viner R. Adolescent development. BMJ 2005;330(7486):301–4.

11. Cauberghe V, Van Wesenbeeck I, De Jans S, et al. How Adolescents Use Social Media to Cope with Feelings of Loneliness and Anxiety during COVID-19 Lockdown. Cyberpsychol, Behav Soc Netw 2021;24(4):250–7.

12. Charmaraman L, Lynch AD, Richer AM, et al. Examining Early Adolescent Positive and Negative Social Technology Behaviors and Well-Being During the COVID-19 Pandemic. tmbapaopenorg 2022;3(1). https://doi.org/10.1037/tmb0000062.

13. Saud M, Mashud M, Ida R. Usage of social media during the pandemic: Seeking support and awareness about COVID-19 through social media platforms. J Publ Aff 2020;20(4). https://doi.org/10.1002/pa.2417.

14. Vaingankar JA. Social Media–Driven Routes to Positive Mental Health Among Youth: Qualitative Enquiry and Concept Mapping Study. JMIR Pediatrics and Parenting 2022;5(1):1–14.

15. Vogels Emily. Teens and cyberbullying 2022. Pew Research Center, Pew Research Center; 2022. Available at: www.pewresearch.org/internet/2022/12/15/teens-and-cyberbullying-2022/.

16. Ofori S, Choongo J, Kekop M, et al. Social Media Usage and Transitioning into Online Classes During COVID- 19-A Survey of Undergraduate Students in Georgia, United States. Int J Educ Dev using Inf Commun Technol (IJEDICT) 2021; 17(4):67–80. Available at: https://files.eric.ed.gov/fulltext/EJ1335759.pdf.

17. Sobaih AEE, Palla IA, Baquee A. Social Media Use in E-Learning amid COVID 19 Pandemic: Indian Students' Perspective. Int J Environ Res Publ Health 2022; 19(9):5380.

18. Hamilton JL, Nesi J, Choukas-Bradley S. Reexamining Social Media and Socio-emotional Well-Being Among Adolescents Through the Lens of the COVID-19 Pandemic: A Theoretical Review and Directions for Future Research. Perspect Psychol Sci 2021;17(3). 174569162110141.

19. Topolovec-Vranic J, Natarajan K. The Use of Social Media in Recruitment for Medical Research Studies: a Scoping Review. J Med Internet Res 2016;18(11):e286.

20. Welch V, Petkovic J, Pardo Pardo J, et al. Interactive social media interventions to promote health equity: an overview of reviews. Health Promotion and Chronic Disease Prevention in Canada : Research, Policy and Practice 2016;36(4):63–75.

21. Marciano L, Ostroumova M, Schulz Peter J, et al. Digital Media Use and Adolescents' Mental Health during the Covid-19 Pandemic: a Systematic Review and Meta-Analysis. Front Public Health 2022;9(793868). https://doi.org/10.3389/fpubh.2021.793868.

22. Magson NR, Freeman JYA, Rapee RM, et al. Risk and Protective Factors for Prospective Changes in Adolescent Mental Health during the COVID-19 Pandemic. J Youth Adolesc 2020;50(1):44–57.

23. Magis-Weinberg L, Gys CL, Berger EL, et al. Positive and Negative Online Experiences and Loneliness in Peruvian Adolescents During the COVID-19 Lockdown. J Res Adolesc 2021;31(3):717–33.

24. I-Hua C, Chen CY, Pakpour AH, et al. Problematic internet-related behaviors mediate the associations between levels of internet engagement and distress among schoolchildren during COVID-19 lockdown: A longitudinal structural equation modeling study. Journal of Behavioral Addictions 2021;10(1). https://doi.org/10.1556/2006.2021.00006.

25. Ellis WE, Dumas TM, Forbes LM. Physically isolated but socially connected: Psychological adjustment and stress among adolescents during the initial COVID-19 crisis. Can J Behav Sci/Rev Can Sci Comport 2020;52(3):177–87.

26. Sherman LE, Payton AA, Hernandez LM, et al. The Power of the Like in Adolescence: Effects of Peer Influence on Neural and Behavioral Responses to Social Media. Psychol Sci 2016;27(7):1027–35.

27. Garthe RC, Kim S, Welsh M, et al. Cyber-Victimization and Mental Health Concerns among Middle School Students Before and During the COVID-19 Pandemic. J Youth Adolesc 2023;52(4):840–51.

28. Cooper M, Reilly EE, Siegel JA, et al. Eating disorders during the COVID-19 pandemic and quarantine: an overview of risks and recommendations for treatment and early intervention. Eat Disord 2022;30(1):54–76. https://doi.org/10.1080/10640266.2020.1790271.

29. Simone M, Emery RL, Hazzard VM, et al. Disordered eating in a population-based sample of young adults during the COVID-19 outbreak. Int J Eat Disord 2021;54(7):1189–201. https://doi.org/10.1002/eat.23505.

30. Nutley SK, Falise AM, Henderson R, et al. Impact of the COVID-19 Pandemic on Disordered Eating Behavior: Qualitative Analysis of Social Media Posts. JMIR Ment Health 2021;8(1):e26011. https://doi.org/10.2196/26011.

31. Zeiler M, Wittek T, Kahlenberg L, et al. Impact of COVID-19 Confinement on Adolescent Patients with Anorexia Nervosa: A Qualitative Interview Study Involving Adolescents and Parents. Int J Environ Res Public Health 2021;18(8):4251. https://doi.org/10.3390/ijerph18084251.

32. Vall-Roqué H, Andrés A, Saldaña C. The impact of COVID-19 lockdown on social network sites use, body image disturbances and self-esteem among adolescent and young women. Prog Neuro Psychopharmacol Biol Psychiatr 2021;110:110293.

33. Silence C, Rice SM, Pollock S, et al. Life After Lockdown: Zooming Out on Perceptions in the Post-Videoconferencing Era. International Journal of Women's Dermatology 2021;7(5Part B). https://doi.org/10.1016/j.ijwd.2021.08.009.

34. Werling A, Walitza S, Grünblatt E, et al. Media use before, during and after COVID-19 lockdown according to parents in a clinically referred sample in child and adolescent psychiatry: Results of an online survey in Switzerland. Compr Psychiatr 2021;109:152260.

35. Akdağ B, Önder A, Gül ME, et al. Online Behavioral Addictions Among Adolescents Before and After the COVID-19 Pandemic. Cureus 2023;15(8):e43231.

36. Anderson M, Jiang J. Teens, social media & technology 2018. Pew Research Center; 2018. Available at: https://www.pewresearch.org/internet/2018/05/31/teens-social-media-technology-2018/.
37. Draženović M, Vukušić Rukavina T, Machala Poplašen L. Impact of Social Media Use on Mental Health within Adolescent and Student Populations during COVID-19 Pandemic: Review. Int J Environ Res Public Health 2023;20(4):3392.

Innovative Strategies for Addressing Adolescent Health in Primary Care Through Telehealth

Elvira Chiccarelli, MD[a],*, Steve North, MD, MPH[b], Ryan H. Pasternak, MD, MPH[c]

KEYWORDS

• Adolescent • Telehealth • Confidentiality • Disparities

KEY POINTS

• While telehealth can be beneficial for promoting health equity among adolescents, each advance is balanced by additional considerations and an evidence-based approach to telehealth implementation in the future will ensure maximum impact on the health of adolescents.
• Efforts to address the digital divide and ensure equal access to telehealth services for all adolescents are critical to achieve health equity goals.
• Addressing structural barriers and social determinants of health that affect adolescents' access to health care remains essential to further improve health equity in contraceptive care.
• The regulatory and funding landscape has not yet consistently evolved in the US health care system to support fully integrated telehealth services. Early successes are encouraging, and perhaps we will one day all be able to simply "call the doctor" again for our care.

INTRODUCTION

On May 11, 2023, US public health officials ended the coronavirus disease 2019 (COVID-19) virus public health emergency (PHE).[1] The crisis has shaped the health care system, physicians, and adolescents alike. In this issue of Pediatric Clinics, the authors focus on how the PHE changed adolescent health care needs. The PHE accelerated adolescent-friendly changes in health care delivery systems. However, to

[a] Brooke Army Medical Center, 3100 Schofield Road, Fort Sam Houston, TX 78234, USA;
[b] Center for Rural Health Innovation, 167 Locust Street, Spruce Pine, NC 28777, USA;
[c] Louisiana State University School of Medicine, Childrens Mercy Kansas City, 3101 Broadway Boulevard, Kansas City, MO 64111, USA
* Corresponding author.
E-mail address: elchica2016@gmail.com

Pediatr Clin N Am 71 (2024) 693–706
https://doi.org/10.1016/j.pcl.2024.04.006
0031-3955/24/Published by Elsevier Inc.

pediatric.theclinics.com

achieve health care equity for adolescents, additional changes are necessary. Telehealth may remedy some of the gaps, while leaving others unaddressed in unanticipated ways. Telehealth, or virtual health, refers to a group of methods by which health care can be provisioned remotely by means of synchronous telecommunications technology. These technologies include not only audio and video components, but increasingly also include the use of smartphone-based applications and remote health monitoring devices.

Telehealth has existed in some form since the invention of telecommunication through the telegraph and the telephone, though development has accelerated with concurrent technological advances. More recently, development of virtual health services emerged as part of Federal requirements for the use of electronic health records. When primary care offices offered limited in-person access in the early PHE, existing practices and new entities rose to the challenge of providing care in new ways. Physicians will recall the rapid evolution of telehealth services facilitated by early changes in reimbursement.[1,2] This delivery of care shows promise in many of the fields specifically discussed in this issue.[3–6] The early PHE changed many prior logistical barriers to telemedicine, most notably with Congressional alterations to Medicare and Medicaid restrictions in March 2020. These alterations added flexibility concerning where telemedicine could originate, improved reimbursement rates, and specified platforms to be used.[2] Additionally, interstate licensing regulations were relaxed and telehealth reimbursement expanded to include multiple allied health professions. Many other state, federal, and private payors followed the example, resulting in a 7.5 times increase in telehealth visits in 2020, compared with prior to the PHE.[2,7] Pediatric patients likely benefitted from the addition of allied health expansions[7] However, some changes were tied to the PHE declaration and may expire in the coming months. It is likely that regulations specific to Health Insurance Portability and Accountability Act (HIPAA) compliance of video telehealth platforms will resume, as well as those for state licensure strictly in the state where the patient is located. The trend in the field of virtual care currently is toward liberalization of restrictions and continued payment for virtual care services.[2,7,8]

Today virtual care continues to be a popular service, with twice the number of clinicians practicing telemedicine today compared with prior to the PHE.[2] Patients consistently rate telehealth as acceptable, or even preferable to traditional care.[9] Multiple professional societies support the use of telehealth for appropriate cases.[10–13] It is essential to note that the availability and regulations surrounding telehealth services, especially contraceptive care, may vary depending on the country, state, or region. In this article, the authors will explore the expansion and implications of telehealth utilization for adolescent-specific concerns.

CLINICAL RELEVANCE
Contraception

Contraception care is a key element of adolescent health in the context of comprehensive sexual health care. Telehealth has had an increasingly important reaching impact in providing this care and promoting health equity of teens in recent years.[14] Services provided include counseling, eligibility screening, initial prescriptions, and refills and this has resulted in improved access to contraception in remote settings.[15] Additionally, telehealth can provide easier access to ongoing contraceptive care including adjustments and method switching.[16] Since long-acting reversible contraception (LARC) cannot be delivered via telehealth, some professionals have expressed concern that patients accessing contraception via telehealth may be less likely to choose an

LARC method; however, this has not been borne out in the literature.[17] Indeed, both LARC and telehealth contraception rates continue to rise in tandem.[18]

Telehealth contraception *can* play a crucial role in addressing health equity for adolescents in several ways, but it has not been the perfect solution. Telehealth allows adolescents to access contraceptive care without the need to travel to a physical clinic.[19] Although it has been previously hypothesized that this would improve health care access to rural areas, multiple studies have shown that telehealth contraceptive care is not more routinely utilized by rural residents.[19] Telehealth consultations offer a level of privacy and confidentiality that may be particularly important for adolescents who may be uncomfortable discussing sensitive topics like contraception in person, yet there are concerns regarding health care data privacy rules with telehealth care.[20] Adolescents facing cultural or societal stigma surrounding sexual health may find telehealth services more appealing as they can seek care discreetly from the privacy of their homes. The authors will discuss confidentiality concerns later.

Obesity

Telehealth can be a valuable tool in addressing obesity in adolescents by providing remote access to health care services, promoting behavioral changes, and supporting ongoing monitoring and management. Appropriate medically supervised management of weight loss through lifestyle change alone includes a standard of care of a minimum 26 patient contact hours annually, and traditionally delivered care currently fails to consistently meet this standard of care.[5] Multiple technological solutions to combat pediatric and adolescent obesity are under investigation with inconclusive findings thus far.[5,21] As our society and medical system now begin to understand obesity as a complex, chronic disease requiring interdisciplinary and subspecialty care, telehealth will be a necessary tool to fight the obesity epidemic. During telehealth consultations for obesity, health care professionals including physicians, counselors, dieticians, and physical therapists discuss the adolescent's weight status, medical history, lifestyle habits, and dietary behaviors and offer personalized guidance, education, and recommendations for managing obesity.[21] The first American Academy of Pediatrics Clinical Practice guidelines released this year recommend that subspecialty level care for the disease of pediatric obesity should be integrated earlier in this disease, and telehealth has the potential to improve the reach of tertiary care for the 1 in 5 children and adolescents nationwide affected by obesity.[22,23] Additionally, virtual health platforms can facilitate behavioral interventions, such as cognitive-behavioral therapy or motivational interviewing, to address emotional eating, stress-related behaviors, and unhealthy coping mechanisms that may contribute to obesity.[24] Multiple weight loss and calorie tracking apps show promise to promote intensive lifestyle change, with randomized controlled trial using it pending for 2024.[25] Mobile health apps also show promise to gather data on physical activity and engage adolescents through text messaging in between appointments.[24,26–30] Finally, telehealth can facilitate collaboration between various health care professionals involved in the management of adolescent obesity, such as pediatricians, dietitians, psychologists, and physical therapists. This coordinated approach ensures comprehensive care tailored to the individual's needs.

Gender Health

Adolescent-specific guidelines and treatment protocols for gender-affirming care emerged in the United States and Europe largely over the last 2 decades.[31] Subsequently, the COVID-19 PHE spurred increased use and acceptance of telehealth for adolescent and young adult gender-affirming care (AYA-GAC).[32–34] Since then, telehealth has emerged as a tool for clinical service delivery that reduces inequities in care and increases access to limited AYA-GAC services.[35] But little had been known about the impact of care on transgender youth or provision of AYA-GAC.

Transgender persons are well known to suffer disproportionate health care risks many of which may be related to societal stigma or limitations in access to care.[35] Given these outcomes, opportunities to reduce barriers to care for these youth and provide AYA-GAC in ways that meet their needs require prioritization. Simultaneously, attention to aspects of telehealth that may exacerbate inequities, such as lack of cellphone, internet, or electricity is needed. The authors discuss more on the equity concerns of telehealth care later. For those patients with access to these commodities, telehealth represents an important opportunity to provide more transgender and gender-diverse youth access to supportive care while reducing common geographic and structural barriers to care. Recent data have shown that adolescent patients desire GAC via telehealth in specialty and primary care settings.[36] Those youth with lower levels of perceived parental support for care were more likely to desire telehealth for AYA-GAC.[33]

Use of telehealth services to support primary care providers' (PCP) provision of AYA-GAC has shown limitations when specialists are using telehealth-based consultation and training platforms for PCPs.[34] Perhaps predictably, these mirror everyday administrative and clinical issues in medicine and include electronic health record, patient portal messaging, and billing integration concerns. Additionally, the legal landscape of telehealth is unique and evolving with respect to clinician's ability to provide AYA-GAC across state lines considering evolving legislation on gender care for minors.[34] While this represents a logistical challenge for health systems, telehealth AYA-GAC may also be a unique opportunity to reach underserved adolescents through creative solutions. For example, a recent study showed that telehealth nursing was effective for injection teaching for gender-affirming hormone therapy (GAHT).[35]

Mental Health & Substance Use Disorders

The field of behavioral health has perhaps most vigorously entered the telehealth space, both due to increasing need in recent years as well as excellent adaptability of this field to virtual care.[37] It is estimated that at the height of the PHE, mental health telehealth expanded by a factor of 20 to 30.[38] The full range of existing face-to-face mental health services is easily adaptable to both videoconferencing and telephonic encounters through multiple web and app-based platforms. In this field, expanding the reach of existing providers remains particularly important in the face of a persistent unmet need for child and adolescent mental health providers.[39] In addition to synchronized provider sessions, mobile and web-based apps to support pediatric mental health exist with more in development. Multiple prominent apps for pediatric behavioral health telehealth have been clinically validated.[40–42] Multiple clinical protocols and trials are underway to further investigate clinical efficacy of telehealth tools for specific chronic and mental health diagnoses for children.[43] While this field is promising, the authors note concerns later regarding limitations of tele-connectivity and confidentiality, both of which are especially pertinent to the delivery of mental health care. Telehealth has also been rated as less acceptable and preferable by both pediatric and rural populations, which raises concerns for efficacy of services to these populations.[44,45] For physicians seeking to learn about app-based mental health platforms, the authors can recommend the American Psychological Association's objective model for mobile health applications.[46]

Substance use treatment is 1 clinical arena which already has a wealth of clinically validated telehealth strategies. Substance use disorders continue to be the highest among young adults aged 18 to 25.[47] The PHE facilitated favorable regulatory changes specific to substance abuse disorder treatment.[48] Prior to 2018, a slew of federal and state regulations as well as reimbursement barriers existed to providing large scale telehealth medications for opioid use disorder.[48,49] The landscape began to shift with the SUPPORT act which allowed tele-prescribing of controlled substances including buprenorphine.[49] With declaration of the PHE the following year, the drug enforcement administration (DEA) further relaxed any requirement for an in-person visit for these medications and allowed audio-only evaluation.[48,49] Multiple states also allowed for decreased licensure requirements and cross-state telehealth practice. In 2020, Substance Abuse and Mental Health Services Administration (SAMHSA) permitted the use of take-home methadone doses of up to 28 days for stable patients.[48] Next in 2021, the HHS reduced barriers to suboxone prescribing by allowing prescription for up to 30 patients per provider without X waiver for this safe and highly effective medication.[48,49] The summation of these changes has resulted in increased substance used disorder treatment, increased research into the field of substance use disorder (SUD) treatment, and increased patient satisfaction with comparable efficacy to previous deliveries of care.[49] This victory is, however, muted in that many of these relaxed regulations and reimbursement practices were tied to the formal PHE declaration. Many, including use of take-home methadone doses, will expire within months of the end of PHE.

Eating Disorders

The COVID-19 PHE spurred with a dramatic unexpected increase in AYA diagnosis of clinical eating disorders, especially those severe enough to require hospitalization.[50,51] Due to obvious logistical constraints on telehealth for physical examination and evaluation, clinicians were concerned if this transition would allow for effective care for eating disorders, particularly for adolescents and young adult patients.

However, since those early months of the PHE, increasing use of and data about telehealth as an integral part of eating disorder treatment has emerged. The mainstay of treatment for restrictive eating disorders is outpatient family-based therapy.[51] This method requires parental involvement and engagement between mental health specialists, patients, and dieticians or nutritional experts in eating disorder care. Given the intensity of this care, telehealth was not widely used for this form of treatment before the PHE.[52,53] Since then, emerging evidence has shown effectiveness and acceptance of this method of clinical care delivery for patients and parents.[52,53]

CARE DELIVERY
School-Based Health Centers

Telehealth has been used to provide care in schools for almost 3 decades and has evolved to provide a broad spectrum of care at schools in urban, rural, and suburban communities.[54,55] Prior to the PHE, the number of schools with access to medical care via telehealth grew faster than the number that gained bricks and mortar school-based health centers.[56] This has been attributed to the lower cost of implementing a school-based telehealth program and the ability to serve students at schools that do not have the volume of students needed to support a bricks and mortar school-based health center.

Telehealth services can range from health education to diagnosis and treatment of medical conditions, and research has shown that students, parents, and school staff report a high degree of satisfaction with telehealth services in schools.[57] School health leaders identify an increased need for mental health services and providing care via telehealth as 2 dominant themes in the evolution of health care a school.[58] By providing access to care at school, school-based telehealth programs eliminate many technological and geographic barriers seen in other telehealth programs.

Providing medical care via telehealth in schools has evolved since its inception and now, using peripherals, the care is often seen as equivalent to that provided during in person care with the benefit of students not needing to leave school.[59] There are many models for staffing a school-based telehealth program. However, the common components of ensuring confidentiality, receiving consent from a parent or guardian as appropriate, and navigating the regulations outlined by HIPAA and Family Educational Rights and Privacy Act (FERPA) remain the priorities in this space.[60] The scope of medical care being provided in schools via telehealth includes asthma care, psychiatry, primary care, and urgent care.

Schools are the site of care for a broad range of health services, not just medical care.[59] Over the past 10 years, school-based teledentistry has grown rapidly and addresses dental issues in underserved communities.[61] School nurses are using telehealth to both connect to medical care but also to provide remote supervision of insulin administration and health education.[62] Occupational therapy identified telehealth to provide mandated services during the PHE and sees it as a way to expand the reach of a limited number of practitioners.[63] Speech and language therapy delivered via telehealth is shown to have an equal impact to that delivered in person.[64] The presence of school-based telemedicine programs reduces absenteeism which adversely impacts graduation and academic achievement.[65] Moving forward, physicians and other health care providers should evaluate the benefits of incorporating care in schools via telemedicine as part of their practice.

Incarcerated Youth

Telehealth has been increasingly used to provide medical and mental health services to incarcerated youth, addressing their health care needs, and promoting overall well-being. In this respect, data support that telehealth is at least as efficacious as face-to-face health care in terms of patient satisfaction and treatment completion.[66] Additionally, telehealth can effectively link incarcerated youth with families for both family therapy and ongoing support, factors shown to improve rates of recidivism and substance use at release.[67]

Telemedicine supports pre-release planning, helping incarcerated youth prepare for their transition back into the community by ensuring they have access to necessary health care services upon release.[68] It is important to note that the availability and extent of telehealth services for incarcerated youth may vary depending on the policies and resources of individual prisons and the legal frameworks in place.

Confidentiality

Studies of telehealth services with adolescents during the COVID-19 PHE demonstrated a small but concerning number of adolescent patients were not able to receive services via telehealth confidentially.[69] Most concerning were cases where patients had to schedule in-person appointments to be able to see providers confidentially and disclose abusive behavior.[70]

That said, for many adolescents, the ability to see a health care provider via telehealth may augment confidentiality by reducing the need to rely on parents or others for transportation, allowing care while parents are at work or attending other duties, and provide care in safe spaces in the home when they exist. Options that have been recommended and used by providers for addressing confidentiality for adolescent telehealth visits when patients are not alone include use of headphones to

Table 1
Selected policy and reimbursement updates for telehealth practice[1,2,7,8,48]

Policy	Agency	Implications	Expiration
Consolidated Appropriations Act of 2022	Medicare	Federally Qualified Health Centers and Rural Health Clinics can serve as a distant site provider for behavioral telehealth services. Medicare patients can receive telehealth services for behavioral health care in their home. There are no geographic restrictions for originating site for behavioral telehealth services. Rural Emergency Hospitals are eligible originating sites for telehealth	Permanent
Notification of Enforcement Discretion for Telehealth	Dept of Health and Human Services	Cessation of relaxed privacy restrictions that temporarily allowed covered providers to use popular communication apps to deliver telehealth during the coronavirus disease 2019 public health emergency	May 11, 2023
Temporary Extension of COVID-19 Telemedicine Flexibilities for Prescription of Controlled Medications (Ryan Haight Act)	Drug Enforcement Agency	Temporarily allows controlled substances to be prescribed without an in-person examination.	November 11, 2024
Consolidated Appropriations Act of 2023	Medicare	An in-person visit within 6 months of an initial behavioral telehealth service, and annually thereafter, is not required. Behavioral telehealth services can be delivered using audio-only communication platforms. Telehealth services can be provided by all eligible Medicare providers	December 31, 2024

prevent questions from being overheard, phrasing yes/no questions, and use of the chat function to allow patients to type responses or questions within the telehealth platform.[70] Despite concerns about the impact of socioeconomic status on access to technology to connect in telehealth visits, this was not seen in this study.[70] Yet, the authors noted that socioeconomic status impacted confidentiality due to "crowded living conditions."[70]

While telehealth expanded significantly during the PHE, other regulatory changes also impacted the flow of confidential information in health care. Enforcement of the 21st Century Cures Act rule prohibiting "information-blocking" went into effect on September 1st, 2023.[71] This rule requires much of the information contained in medical records to be shared with patients and designated proxies[71–73]

While telehealth may provide adolescents with some private access to medical visits without parental knowledge, broad concerns exist regarding the ability to ensure access to confidential adolescent health care services and comply with these aforementioned rules.[73] More specifically, the relationship between telehealth services and the Act has not been extensively explored. By providing access to care at school, school-based telehealth programs eliminate many technological and geographic barriers seen in other telehealth programs. Providing medical care via telehealth in schools has evolved since its inception and now, using peripherals, the care is often seen as equivalent to that provided during in person care with the benefit of students not needing to leave school.[59]

Equity

Virtual care is often cited as a proposed tool to improve inequities in health care by expanding access to rural locations, or patients who lack transportation or resources to attend appointments.[59] These issues as well as those concerning confidentiality are of particular importance to adolescents. Unfortunately, the body of evidence surrounding the actual impact of virtual care in these areas is weak. For example, telehealth services can include interpreters or translation services, but many current platforms are not readily used for this purpose.[74]

Additionally, in truly rural areas, access to broadband connectivity to support virtual health is significantly lacking such that telehealth services do not reach any more population than traditional care otherwise would[75–77] In urban areas, people from minoritized racial/ethnic groups comprise 75% of those without broadband connectivity.[76] Studies of telehealth utilization likewise do not demonstrate consistent utilization trends among minoritized groups or lesbian, gay, bisexual, transgender, and queer patients who stand to benefit the most from virtual health care.[78,79] This may be due to implementation problems, but it may also be indicative of larger advocacy trends which lack appropriate stakeholder inputs in designing systems of care. Either way, it is time that those responsible for implementing telehealth initiatives take a more evidence-based approach in supporting rural youth and youth from minoritized groups.

SUMMARY

While telehealth can be beneficial for promoting health equity among adolescents, each advance is balanced by additional considerations and an evidence-based approach to telehealth implementation in the future will ensure maximum impact on the health of adolescents. Efforts to address the digital divide and ensure equal access to telehealth services for all adolescents are critical to achieve health equity goals. Additionally, addressing structural barriers and social determinants of health that affect adolescents' access to health care remains essential to further improve health equity in contraceptive care. Finally, the regulatory and funding landscape has not yet consistently evolved in the US health care system to support fully integrated telehealth services. Early successes are encouraging, and perhaps we will 1 day all be able to simply "call the doctor" again for our care.

CLINICS CARE POINTS

- Telehealth (or virtual health) refers to a group of methods of health care delivery by which health care can be provisioned remotely using synchronous communication technology or remote health monitoring devices.
- Current adolescent-specific issues well served by virtual health platforms include contraception, obesity, gender-affirming care, mental health, and eating disorders.
- Special considerations exist for the delivery of telehealth-based care in school-based health centers and care for incarcerated youth, and with the interest of promoting confidentiality and health equity.
- Providers should be aware of a changing regulatory landscape regarding telehealth restriction and reimbursement (**Table 1**).

DISCLOSURE

The authors have no relevant financial or non-financial relationships to disclose relating to the content of this activity. The views expressed in this presentation are those of the author and do not necessarily reflect the official policy or position of the Department of Defense, the United States Air Force, or the US Government.

REFERENCES

1. "End of the Federal COVID-19 Public Health Emergency (PHE) Declaration." Centers for Disease Control and Prevention, Centers for Disease Control and Prevention. Available at: www.cdc.gov/coronavirus/2019-ncov/your-health/end-of-phe.html#: ~ :text=May%2011%2C%202023%2C%20marks%20the,to%20the% 20COVID%2D19%20pandemic. [Accessed 28 September 2023].
2. Telehealth policy changes after the COVID-19 public health emergency. telehealth.hhs.gov, Available at: https://telehealth.hhs.gov/providers/telehealth-policy/policy-changes-after-the-covid-19-public-health-emergency#: ~ :text=The %20Administration%27s%20plan%20is%20to,emergency%20through%20December %2031%2C%202024. (Accessed 1 October 2023).
3. Gorrell S, Reilly, Brosof, et al. Use of telehealth in the management of adolescent eating disorders: patient perspectives and future directions suggested from the COVID-19 pandemic. Adolesc Health Med Ther 2022;13:45–53.
4. Cantor J, McBain, Kofner, et al. Telehealth adoption by mental health and substance use disorder treatment facilities in the COVID-19 pandemic. Psychiatr Serv 2022;73(4):411–7.
5. Fitch AK, Bays HE. Obesity definition, diagnosis, bias, standard operating procedures (SOPs), and telehealth: An Obesity Medicine Association (OMA) Clinical Practice Statement (CPS) 2022. Obes Pillars 2022;1:100004.
6. Cantor AG, Nelson, Pappas, et al. Telehealth for Women's Preventive Services for Reproductive Health and Intimate Partner Violence: a Comparative Effectiveness Review. J Gen Intern Med 2023;38(7):1735–43.

7. Pandya A, Waller W, Portnoy JM. The regulatory environment of telemedicine after COVID-19. J Allergy Clin Immunol Pract 2022;10(10):2500–5.

8. Shaver J. The state of telehealth before and after the COVID-19 pandemic. Prim Care 2022;49(4):517–30.

9. Hays RD, Skootsky AS. Patient experience with in-person and telehealth visits before and during the COVID-19 pandemic at a large integrated health system in the United States. J Gen Intern Med 2022;37(4):847–52.

10. Vimalananda VG, Brito, Eiland, et al. Appropriate use of telehealth visits in endocrinology: policy perspective of the endocrine society. The Journal of Clinical Endocrinology & Metabolism 2022;107(11):2953–62.

11. Chen A, Ayub MH, Mishuris RG, et al. Telehealth Policy, Practice, and Education: a Position Statement of the Society of General Internal Medicine. J Gen Intern Med 2023;1–8.

12. Franciosi JP, Berg, Rosen, et al. North American Society for Pediatric Gastroenterology, Hepatology, and Nutrition Position Statement for Telehealth. J Pediatr Gastroenterol Nutr 2023;76(5):684–94.

13. Keder RD, Mittal, Stringer, et al. Society for developmental & behavioral pediatrics position statement on telehealth. J Dev Behav Pediatr 2022;43(1):55–9.

14. Lindberg LD, Mueller, Haas, et al. Telehealth for contraceptive care during the COVID-19 pandemic: Results of a 2021 national survey. Am J Public Health 2022;112(S5):S545–54.

15. Sundstrom B, DeMaria, Ferrara, et al. "The closer, the better:" the role of telehealth in increasing contraceptive access among women in rural South Carolina. Matern Child Health J 2019;23(9):1196–205.

16. Song B, Boulware, Wong, et al. "This has definitely opened the doors": Provider perceptions of patient experiences with telemedicine for contraception in Illinois. Perspect Sex Reprod Health 2022;54(3):80–9.

17. Durante JC, Sims, Jarin, et al. Long-Acting Reversible Contraception for Adolescents: A Review of Practices to Support Better Communication, Counseling, and Adherence. Adolesc Health Med Ther 2023;14:97–114.

18. Mueller J, VandeVusse, Sackietey, et al. Effects of the COVID-19 pandemic on publicly supported clinics providing contraceptive services in four US states. Contraception X 2023;5:100096.

19. Rao L, Comfort, Dojiri, et al. Telehealth for contraceptive services during the COVID-19 pandemic: provider perspectives. Wom Health Issues 2022;32(5):477–83.

20. Watzlaf VJM, Zhou, Dealmeida, et al. A systematic review of research studies examining telehealth privacy and security practices used by healthcare providers. Int J Telerehabil 2017;9(2):39–59.

21. Fowler LA, Grammer, Staiano, et al. Harnessing technological solutions for childhood obesity prevention and treatment: a systematic review and meta-analysis of current applications. Int J Obes 2021;45(5):957–81.

22. Hampl SE, Hassink, Skinner, et al. Executive Summary: Clinical Practice Guideline for the Evaluation and Treatment of Children and Adolescents With Obesity. Pediatrics 2023;151(2):e2022060640.

23. "Childhood Obesity Facts." Centers for Disease Control and Prevention, Centers for Disease Control and Prevention, Available at: www.cdc.gov/obesity/data/childhood.html#:~:text=For%20children%20and%20adolescents%20aged,to%2019%2Dyear%2Dolds, (Accessed 1 October 2023), 2022.

24. Cardel MI, Atkinson, Taveras, et al. Obesity treatment among adolescents: a review of current evidence and future directions. JAMA Pediatr 2020;174(6): 609–17.
25. Ufholz K, Bhargava D. A review of telemedicine interventions for weight loss. Current Cardiovascular Risk Reports 2021;15:1–9.
26. Fang Y-Y, Lee, Wu, et al. Effect of a novel telehealth device for dietary cognitive behavioral intervention in overweight or obesity care. Sci Rep 2023;13(1):6441.
27. Myers RE, Medvedev, Oh, et al. A Randomized Controlled Trial of a Telehealth Family-Delivered Mindfulness-Based Health Wellness (MBHW) Program for Self-Management of Weight by Adolescents with Intellectual and Developmental Disabilities. Mindfulness 2023;14(3):524–37.
28. Chin SO, Keum, Woo, et al. Successful weight reduction and maintenance by using a smartphone application in those with overweight and obesity. Sci Rep 2016; 6(1):34563.
29. Sysko R, Bibeau, Boyar, et al. A 2.5-Year Weight Management Program Using Noom Health: Protocol for a Randomized Controlled Trial. JMIR Res Protoc 2022;11(8):e37541.
30. Vajravelu ME, Arslanian S. Mobile health and telehealth interventions to increase physical activity in adolescents with obesity: a promising approach to engaging a hard-to-reach population. Current Obesity Reports 2021;1–9.
31. Carswell JM, Lopez L, Rosenthal SM. The Evolution of Adolescent Gender-Affirming Care: An Historical Perspective. Horm Res Paediatr 2022;95(6):649–56.
32. Stoehr JR, Hamidian Jahromi, Hunter, et al. Telemedicine for Gender-Affirming Medical and Surgical Care: A Systematic Review and Call-to-Action. Transgend Health 2022;7(2):117–26.
33. Sequeira GM, Kidd, Coulter, et al. Transgender youths' perspectives on telehealth for delivery of gender-affirming care. J Adolesc Health 2021;68(6):1207–10.
34. Sequeira GM, Kahn, Bocek, et al. Pediatric Primary Care Providers' Perspectives on Telehealth Platforms to Support Care for Transgender and Gender-Diverse Youths: Exploratory Qualitative Study. JMIR Hum Factors 2023;10(1):e39118.
35. Johns MM, Lowry, Andrzejewski, et al. "Transgender Identity and Experiences of Violence Victimization, Substance Use, Suicide Risk, and Sexual Risk Behaviors Among High School Students - 19 States and Large Urban School Districts, 2017, 2017.". MMWR Morb Mortal Wkly Rep 2019;68(3):67–71.
36. Nightingale KJ, Jelinek SK, Jones C, et al. 19. Telehealth versus in-person instruction for adolescents and young adults initiating gender-affirming testosterone therapy. J Adolesc Health 2024;74(3). https://doi.org/10.1016/j.jadohealth.2023. 11.216.
37. "Telemedicine and Telehealth." HealthIT.Gov, Available at: www.healthit.gov/topic/health-it-health-care-settings/public-health/telemedicine-and-telehealth, (Accessed 1 October 2023), 2023.
38. Bestsennyy O, Gilbert G, Harris A, et al. Telehealth: a quarter-trillion-dollar post-COVID-19 reality. New York, NY: McKinsey & Company; 2021. p. 9.
39. McBain RK, Kofner, Stein, et al. Growth and distribution of child psychiatrists in the United States: 2007–2016. Pediatrics 2019;144.
40. Whiteside SPH, Biggs, Tiede, et al. An Online- and Mobile-Based Application to Facilitate Exposure for Childhood Anxiety Disorders. Cogn Behav Pract 2019; 26(3):478–91.
41. Weekly T, Walker, Beck, et al. A review of apps for calming, relaxation, and mindfulness interventions for pediatric palliative care patients. Children 2018;5(2):16.

42. Cunningham NR, Ely, Barber Garcia, et al. Addressing pediatric mental health using telehealth during coronavirus disease-2019 and beyond: A narrative review. Acad Pediatr 2021;21(7):1108–17.

43. Cunningham NR, Kalomiris, Peugh, et al. Cognitive Behavior Therapy Tailored to Anxiety Symptoms Improves Pediatric Functional Abdominal Pain Outcomes: A Randomized Clinical Trial. J Pediatr 2021;230:62.e3.

44. Mseke EP, Jessup B, Barnett T. A systematic review of the preferences of rural and remote youth for mental health service access: Telehealth versus face-to-face consultation. Aust J Rural Health 2023;31(3):346–60.

45. Hoffnung G, Feigenbaum, Schechter, et al. Children and telehealth in mental healthcare: what we have learned from COVID-19 and 40,000+ sessions. Psychiatr Res Clin Pract 2021;3(3):106–14.

46. "Mental Health Apps." Psychiatry.Org - Mental Health Apps. Available at: www.psychiatry.org/psychiatrists/practice/mental-health-apps. [Accessed 28 September 2023].

47. Substance Abuse and Mental Health Services Administration. Key substance use and mental health indicators in the United States: Results from the 2019 national Survey on Drug Use and health (HHS Publication No. PEP20-07-01-001, NSDUH Series H-55). Rockville, MD: Center for Behavioral Health Statistics and Quality, Substance Abuse and Mental Health Services Administration; 2020. Available at: https://www.samhsa.gov/data/.

48. "Laws and Regulations." SAMHSA, Available at: www.samhsa.gov/about-us/who-we-are/laws-regulations#:~:text=SUPPORT%20Act,the%20nation's%20opioid%20overdose%20epidemic. Accessed 1 October. 2023.

49. LaGrotta C, Collins C. Telemedicine and Medication-Assisted Treatment for Opioid Use Disorder. Technology-Assisted Interventions for Substance Use Disorders 2023;13–21.

50. Schwartz MD, Costello LC. Eating disorder in teens during the COVID-19 pandemic. Journal of adolescent health 2021;68(5):1022.

51. Krewson C. Assistant Editor. "Eating Disorder Admissions Increased during COVID-19 Pandemic." Contemporary Pediatrics, Contemporary Pediatrics. 2022. Available at: www.contemporarypediatrics.com/view/eating-disorder-admissions-increased-during-covid-19-pandemic.

52. Steinberg D, Perry, Freestone, et al. Effectiveness of delivering evidence-based eating disorder treatment via telemedicine for children, adolescents, and youth. Eat Disord 2023;31(1):85–101.

53. Levinson CA, Spoor, Keshishian, et al. Pilot outcomes from a multidisciplinary telehealth versus in-person intensive outpatient program for eating disorders during versus before the Covid-19 pandemic. Int J Eat Disord 2021;54(9):1672–9.

54. Whitten PS, Cook DJ. School-based telemedicine: Using technology to bring health care to inner-city children. J Telemed Telecare 1999;5(1_suppl):S23–5.

55. Miller TW, Miller JM. Telemedicine: new directions for health care delivery in Kentucky schools. J Ky Med Assoc 1999;97(4):170–2.

56. Love HE, Schlitt J, Soleimanpour S, et al. Twenty Years Of School-Based Health Care Growth And Expansion. Health Aff 2019;38(5):755–64.

57. Sanchez D, Reiner JF, Sadlon R, et al. Systematic Review of School Telehealth Evaluations. J Sch Nurs 2019;35(1):61–76.

58. Miller K, Goddard A, Cushing K. Exploratory Qualitative Focus Group Analysis of School-based Health Center Policy Issues: Insights From State Leaders. J Pediatr Health Care 2023;37(6):626–35.

59. Ward MM, Merchant KAS, Ullrich F, et al. Telehealth Services for Primary Care and Urgent Care to Support Rural Schools and Students. Telemedicine and e-Health 2023;29(7):1027–34.
60. Garber K, Wells E, Hale KC, et al. Connecting Kids to Care: Developing a School-Based Telehealth Program. J Nurse Pract 2021;17(3):273–8.
61. Kohli R, Clemens J, Mann L, et al. Training dental hygienists to place interim therapeutic restorations in a school-based teledentistry program: Oregon's virtual dental home. J Public Health Dent 2022;82(2):229–38.
62. Marrapese B, Gormley JM, Deschene K. Reimagining School Nursing: Lessons Learned From a Virtual School Nurse. NASN Sch Nurse 2021;36(4):218–25.
63. Abbott-Gaffney C, Jacobs K. Telehealth in school-based practice: Perceived viability to bridge global OT practitioner shortages prior to COVID-19 global health emergency. Work 2020;67(1):29–35.
64. Langbecker DH, Caffery L, Taylor M, et al. Impact of school-based allied health therapy via telehealth on children's speech and language, class participation and educational outcomes. J Telemed Telecare 2019;25(9):559–65.
65. Komisarow S, Hemelt SW. School-Based Healthcare and Absenteeism: Evidence from Telemedicine. SSRN Electron J 2023. https://doi.org/10.2139/ssrn. 4323736.
66. Tian EJ, Venugopalan, Kumar, et al. The impacts of and outcomes from telehealth delivered in prisons: A systematic review. PLoS One 2021;16(5):e0251840.
67. Tolou-Shams M, Bath, McPhee, et al. Juvenile Justice, Technology and Family Separation: A Call to Prioritize Access to Family-Based Telehealth Treatment for Justice-Involved Adolescents' Mental Health and Well-Being. Front Digit Health 2022;4:867366.
68. Brantley AD, Page, Zack, et al. Making the connection: using videoconferencing to increase linkage to care for incarcerated persons living with HIV post-release. AIDS Behav 2019;23(Suppl 1):32–40.
69. Barney A, Buckelew, Mesheriakova, et al. The COVID-19 pandemic and rapid implementation of adolescent and young adult telemedicine: challenges and opportunities for innovation. J Adolesc Health 2020;67(2):164–71.
70. Perry Martha F. Confidential Telehealth Care for Adolescents: Challenges and Solutions Identified During the COVID-19 Pandemic. Curr Pediatr Rep 2023;1–8.
71. "Information Blocking." HHS, 5 July 2023, oig, Available at: hhs.gov/reports-and-publications/featured-topics/information-blocking/, (Accessed 1 October 2023).
72. Act, Century Cures. "interoperability, information blocking, and the ONC health IT certification program.". Fed Regist 2020;85.
73. Pasternak RH, Alderman EM, English A. 21st Century Cures Act ONC Rule: Implications for Adolescent Care and Confidentiality Protections. Pediatrics 2023; 151(Suppl 1).
74. Crawford A, Serhal E. Digital Health Equity and COVID-19: The Innovation Curve Cannot Reinforce the Social Gradient of Health. J Med Internet Res 2020;22(6): e19361.
75. "Broadband Is the Achilles' Heel of Telehealth." Healthcare IT News. 2021. Available at: www.healthcareitnews.com/blog/broadband-achilles-heel-telehealth.
76. White-Williams C, Liu, Shang, et al. Use of telehealth among racial and ethnic minority groups in the United States before and during the COVID-19 pandemic. Public Health Rep 2023;138(1):149–56.
77. Pandit AA, Mahashabde RV, Brown CC, et al. Association between broadband capacity and telehealth utilization among Medicare Fee-for-service beneficiaries

during the COVID-19 pandemic. J Telemed Telecare 2023. https://doi.org/10.1177/1357633X231166026. 1357633X231166026.

78. Mahtta D, Daher M, Lee MT, et al. Promise and perils of telehealth in the current era. Curr Cardiol Rep 2021;23:1–6.

79. Tabler J, Schmitz, Charak, et al. Forgone care among LGBTQ and non-LGBTQ Americans during the COVID-19 pandemic: the role of health, social support, and pandemic-related stress. South Med J 2022;115(10):752–9.

Productive Messaging to Promote Youth Mental Well-Being and Positive Development in Clinical and Advocacy Settings

Merrian J. Brooks, DO, MS[a,b,c,*], Nat Kendall-Taylor, PhD[d],
Kenneth R. Ginsburg, MD, MSEd[a,b,e]

KEYWORDS

- Framing • Health communication • Adolescent development
- Professional development • Role of parent

KEY POINTS

- The current 'crisis narrative' related to youth mental health has 3 key features: (1) It frames youth mental illness as one of dire crisis and utmost urgency; (2) It positions individual effort and choice as the cause and solution to youth mental health challenges; and (3) It "others" those youth with mental illness and plays on stereotypes.
- Individualism, fatalism, and 'othering' are cognitive biases that are evoked when youth mental health communication involves crisis messaging. These cognitive biases can make our communication ineffective.
- These biases and their harmful effects can be overcome using supportive narratives with reframed communication that is rooted in contextualism, pragmatism, efficiency, and collectivism.
- Thoughtful communication rooted in the science-backed approaches described is relevant in all interactions including those with patients/adolescents, parents/caregivers, and the public at large.

BACKGROUND
Introduction

The coronavirus disease 2019 pandemic has had a profound impact on the emotional and mental well-being of young people. There has been a surge of public messaging

Financial disclosure: The authors have indicated they have no financial relationships relevant to this article to disclose.
[a] Craig Dalsimer Division of Adolescent Medicine, Children's Hospital of Philadelphia, 3400 Civic Center Boulevard, Philadelphia, PA 19104, USA; [b] Department of Pediatrics, University of Pennsylvania Perelman School of Medicine; [c] Lead Pediatrician Botswana UPENN Partnership, 214 Independence Avenue, Gaborone, Botswana; [d] FrameWorks Institute, 1333 H Street NW, Washington, DC 20005, USA; [e] Center for Parent and Teen Communication, 2716 South Street, Floor 9, Philadelphia, PA 19146, USA
* Corresponding author.
E-mail address: brooksm2@chop.edu

Pediatr Clin N Am 71 (2024) 707–727
https://doi.org/10.1016/j.pcl.2024.04.009   **pediatric.theclinics.com**
0031-3955/24/© 2024 Elsevier Inc. All rights reserved, including those for text and data mining, AI training, and similar technologies.

efforts designed to raise awareness and advocate for resources to address youth mental health. Pediatric professionals may be using some of these same messages in clinical and advocacy settings when trying to support young people and their families.

While well intentioned, are these messages doing what they are designed to do? Are the narratives pediatric professionals and others are advancing helping to create the social, community, and service changes necessary to address issues of youth mental health and improve well-being, or are these narratives doing harm? And, if the current narrative is undermining the well-being of adolescents or their families, are there alternate ways of framing these issues that build awareness and increase demand for solutions?

Framing is how we present information when we are trying to communicate with youth families and communities; to communicate support, encouragement, or to convince. Effective communication is the cornerstone of pediatric practice. To maximize our messaging around youth mental well-being, we need to take a close look at the narrative that is being advanced, examine the consequences of these ways of framing the issue, and—importantly—use evidence-informed strategies to engage caring adults and move youth mental health and emotional well-being squarely onto the public's agenda. Communication strategies must build demand for the kinds of policies and practices that better address mental health challenges while simultaneously supporting positive youth development and indeed, thriving.

The current narrative on youth mental health has 3 key features that create a 'crisis narrative: (1) It frames the issue as one of dire crisis and utmost urgency; (2) It positions individual effort and choice (young people and caregivers) as the cause of mental health challenges and the solution to the current crisis; and (3) It presents young people dealing with mental health challenges as "other" and plays on stereotypes of young people and other marginalized groups.

While this can increase resources being made available to address youth mental health, this 'crisis narrative' inadvertently perpetuates harmful mindsets and misconceptions about adolescence. This not only affects the way society and parents view adolescents but also how adolescents perceive themselves. While there are undoubtedly many young people experiencing mental health challenges, crisis messaging implies that all adolescents are suffering and underplays those youth who are displaying resilience even in the face of significant challenges. The repercussions of this crisis narrative can be far reaching and long lasting as it reinforces the deficit model of youth.[1] The narrative being advanced sets the context and determines the ground on which our social, policy, and practice decisions will be made for years to come.

As resources are channeled in directions consistent with the current narrative, there is a risk that we may be neglecting tried-and-true solutions: Activating family engagement with evidence-informed parenting practices, highlighting the power of community involvement in the lives of youth, and investing in what we have learned contribute to positive youth development. Here, the authors review some of the pitfalls of the current narrative and provide a practical guide for what pediatric professionals can do to reframe the conversation on adolescent mental health through interactions with youth and families and in communications with policy makers and other stakeholders.

NATURE OF THE PROBLEM
Why the Current Narrative Backfires

The current crisis narrative can promote cognitive shortcuts that can result in inaction and undermine positive youth development. These cognitive shortcuts are cultural mindsets:[1] unconscious, highly shared patterns of reasoning that shape how we see the world and act in it. Seeing how this narrative activates these 3 mindsets and what these mindsets do to our thinking helps us understand both the need to shift from this narrative as well as the features of a more productive one.[2]

The first of these mindsets is individualism. This is the idea that the world is the way that it is because of how hard people try, the decisions they make, the effort they do (or do not) choose to exert, and their application of internal fortitude and willpower. It is not that individualism is wrong; individual drive and choice do matter. The problem is when individualism is the dominant way of seeing the world; if the cause of all problems is failure of individual will, then the only solution is trying harder. This is a dangerous perspective on youth mental health and emotional well-being.

This way of thinking heaps responsibility for mental health challenges onto the backs of young people and lets society and its decisions and policies off the hook. It focuses our attention on better decisions and more effort as the only viable answers to problems, which blocks out the importance of resources, supports, and relationships in understanding the cause of social problems and as key parts of addressing them. Overactive individualism keeps people from seeing that what surrounds us shapes us and casts youth mental health as a *personal trouble* rather than a *public issue*. The current narrative lacks the context necessary for understanding the challenges young adults face, leading to misconceptions and victim blaming.

The second mindset that the current narrative activates is fatalism—the sense that the world is too broken and that the issues we face are too numerous, too big, and too dire to do anything about. When asked to think and engage on yet *another* issue, this mindset leads people to tune out and disengage.

On youth mental health, fatalism makes it hard to motivate action. When something is seen as yet another existential threat, it has become hard to invest a lot of our time and attention in figuring out what can be done. Somewhat ironically, we believe that attempts to appeal to fatalism—the "youth mental health crisis"—may raise awareness of the issue, while backfiring by making the problem that people are now more aware of, seem unsolvable. Rather than focusing on solutions, a crisis-focused narrative steers attention away from the most effective approaches: activating families to harness their support systems and investing in positive youth development.

Finally, "otherism" is the proclivity to see the world in zero-sum terms, where more for one group, by definition, means less for another. Looking at the world in this way, people see a set of warring factions, with competing rather than common interests.

When we see young people as "other"—something our public discourse has made it very easy to do—it is hard to see that we have a stake in their problems. This is especially true when talking about specific groups of young people, those who have been systemically and historically excluded from opportunities and left without the support from which others benefit. If young people are other and this is "their" issue, then it is hard to build broad public engagement or to see the value of using public resources to address this issue. We might raise fear about the issue through othering, but this only reinforces stigma and contributes to negative stereotypes that affect how both society and adolescents see themselves. The myths and misconceptions being reinforced through the current narrative include beliefs that adolescents do not care about engaging with or being guided by adults, are inherently irrational and cannot be reasoned with, are dangerous risk-takers, and are selfish and driven solely by emotions.

These 3 mindsets come together to create the sense that adults should stand aside and that adolescence is an inevitably negative and risky phase that we can just hope to make it through. This takeaway ignores that many adolescents are doing well and the fact that nurturant adult guidance is critical for positive adolescent development.

However, the greatest harm of these mindsets may be the way they overwhelm caregivers and discourage the unwavering presence and guidance that are central to adolescent well-being.

How We Inadvertently Activate These Mindsets

The problem is not just that these mindsets exist but that the dominant narrative and so much of the communications on the issue inadvertently activate these ways of thinking.[3]

Individualism can often be inadvertently promoted in our attempts to encourage patients. For example, every story we hear where perseverance is the reason why a young person experiences a positive outcome activates individualism. Every time the answer to a mental health problem is one individual who, against all odds, succeeds, individualism is strengthened and our focus comes off of systems and supports and onto greater effort, trying harder and making better decisions as the solution to all problems.

Our sense of fatalism is fed every time we hear about the "youth mental health *crisis*" or are presented with a slew of dire statistics about the prevalence and severity of the problem without any mention of solutions. Every time we hear messages focused exclusively on mental health *problems* without any mention of mental *health,* well-being, or resilience, we are sent an invitation to think that building mental *health* is a fool's errand. And every time we see images such as those in **Fig. 1**, we receive a powerful message of hopelessness and isolation—of an issue too big to solve and too impossible to engage with.

Every time we talk about young people as vulnerable, we activate otherism and dampen public support for policies designed to support them. Every message that we receive where young people are without agency—where they are objects that things happen to rather than active characters and participants—our sense of otherism is activated. We are reminded that young people are them, not us.

Taken together, the current narrative results in the following:[4]

- It paralyzes adult action by focusing on the immensity of the problem without being given strategies to solve it.

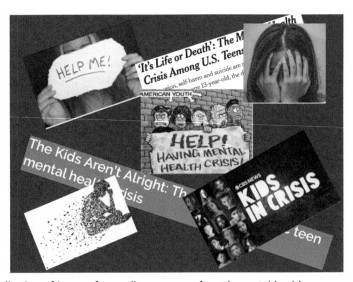

Fig. 1. Collection of images for media coverage of youth mental health.

- It perpetuates damaging stereotypes of teens and paints the generation with a broad brush of brokenness, channeling the way people see young people and the way young people see themselves.
- It diverts attention from the power of investments in positive youth development by focusing all attention on fixing problems.
- It specifically reinforces undermining and incorrect stereotypes that adolescents (as others) do not care what adults think and dislike their parents, that by the time adolescence comes around a young person's development is on autopilot and does not need much input, that adolescents are wired for risk and driven by emotion, and that it is therefore impossible to talk sense into them.

The Dimensions of a Different Story

Pediatric professionals play a central role in reframing these messages to promote meaningful change and can do so using evidence-based communication strategies. Each of these mindsets has an alternative way of thinking that people also have access to. The choices in issue framing have the power to push the unproductive mindsets into the background and pull forward effective ways of thinking.[5]

The counterbalancing mindset of individualism is contextualism, the idea that what surrounds us shapes us. When this mindset is active, people see the importance of public policies, community resources, and social supports and the role they play in enabling or constraining individual will and choice.

The contextualism mindset is cued when community and context are characters in stories that explain the deeper causes of mental health issues and what can happen when those issues are addressed. Examples of efforts that have changed context and resulted in improved youth mental health outcomes are powerful ways of cuing this mindset. For instance, you might note that messages of divisiveness in the community lead to lowered rates of adolescents' sense of belonging and that including adolescents in solution-building enhances their understanding that they can contribute to a cohesive community. In contrast, if a message allows people to walk away thinking that lack of effort is the cause and that more effort is the answer, it has failed to activate "what surrounds us shapes us" thinking. We undermine the productive mindset every time "choose" and "decide" are the most powerful verbs in the stories we hear by underscoring that willpower is really what it's all about.

The counterbalancing mindset of fatalism is pragmatism and efficacy, the sense that we can solve problems. Messages that balance the urgency of a situation with a sense that we can do things to make it better activate pragmatism. Stories of solutions that work and explanations of how action creates better outcomes are other powerful ways of activating this mindset, as are historical examples that show when a community or nation has solved problems and made things better for its people. In simplest terms, every time we underscore the power of supportive adults in young lives, we remind people there is a pragmatic approach that supports youth well-being.

The counterbalancing mindset of otherism is collectivism—the notion of "we." Putting young people in active roles and showing them as people with ideas, agency, and concerns that we all have pulls forward this collective thinking. Deliberately avoiding words that have become common parts of the youth mental health discussion— such as *vulnerable* and *at risk*—also sidesteps the otherism trap. Focusing on the characteristics of the challenge rather than of the people who experience it can help people adopt a more collective mindset. For example, you might say "This young person has been put in an at-risk situation by_____." This construction places the burden on the context where it belongs rather than on the youth. Collectivism is also cued when a set of values—interdependence and common good—are used to frame messages and ground communications. These values counter the tendency to distance and differentiate when it comes to youth mental health.

CLINICS CARE POINTS
The Role of Pediatric Caregivers in Advancing a New, More Productive Narrative

We can break out of the current narrative by shifting from a crisis of mental *ill* health to a focus on positive well-being and mental *health*. To be clear, we do this while simultaneously obtaining needed services for those youth who need focused attention.

Who better than pediatric professionals to generate a productive narrative? Such a narrative would highlight young people as they need to be seen. It would describe their strengths and their temperaments rather than focusing on mistakes they may have made.[6-8] Some of us have known these dynamic individuals their whole lives, which gives us an opportunity to hold on to those people in our minds and reaffirm our commitment to their optimal development. As pediatric professionals prepare for appointments with patients, it means remembering the resilience that young people show in navigating a challenging and unsupportive world. It means rejecting the myths and instead affirming with ourselves, our practice staff, and our colleagues that adolescence is a time of important development that requires experimentation and healthy risk-taking, leaving the comfort zone. When things are going well, it is important to remind young people of the practices that promote well-being. Reminding parents that birth to 5 years of age and 10 to 25 years of age are times of dynamic growth and development can help families remember the importance of supporting positive development.[9] Critically, we empower parents by reminding them of how much they matter to their adolescents every day and how protective it is for them to "stand by teens" in moments of crisis.[10]

As pediatric professionals reframe their own mindsets to shape their approach to young people, they should encourage all staff to do the same. They can stand by young people by reminding the members of their practice that they matter in creating a health sanctuary for all the families and young people they serve. The warmth, empathy, supportiveness, and positivity that young people receive when they enter a clinical setting reassure them that they made the right choice in seeking care.

The American Academy of Pediatrics recommends that pediatric professionals be equipped to manage primary care mental health, which includes using our skills as developmental experts to recognize depression and anxiety in youth. It means understanding which medications are safe in using them. It means using the relationship that we have with patients, strengthening them no matter the young person's mental state, and providing a safe space if any needs do come up. It means when we do need to refer to mental health professionals, we remind adolescents and their families that we continue to be there and that we stand with them.

This reframing of how pediatric professionals think about their work provides the foundation they can work from as they communicate in new and more effective ways with youth and their families, communities, and decision-makers about mental well-being. See **Tables 1–5** for example statements that cue productive versus unproductive thinking.

DISCUSSION
Communicating with Young People About Providing Services and Support

While we often think about communication strategies for large audiences, one-on-one communication with patients and families also requires the thoughtful use of framing. When a young person does need mental health treatment, framing should focus on

Table 1

When speaking with a young person about providing services and support

Say This	Why This Cues Productive Thoughts	Avoid Saying This	Why This Cues Unproductive Thoughts
You deserve support, and we can work together to get you through this challenging time.	The framing conveys a clear sense of efficacy—that there are things that can be done and that the young person plays a role in these things. This is an antidote to the feelings of fatalism and hopelessness that attach to this issue. The use of "we" is a clear cue that this does not all fall to the young person. "Extra support" is an additive frame, avoiding the sense that the young person is lacking skills and resources and instead conveys the sense that the support builds on and supplements existing internal resources the young person possesses. Finally, "deserve" implies an inherent strength—people who have experienced shame need to know that they deserve attention. Importantly, although the term is appropriate and effective in a clinical setting, it should be avoided in community and advocacy settings, where "deserve" invites people to evaluate the worthiness of groups of people and cues individualistic (and racist) bootstrap thinking about who does—and	You really need help, and it is critical you get it right now.	This approach reinforces the deficit model. It suggests an absence of internal resources and may cue the perception that another person rather than the youth holds the solutions. It is also strong on urgency and crisis and lacks any sense of efficacy or agency, which may overwhelm and lead to disengagement.

(continued on next page)

Table 1
(continued)

Say This	Why This Cues Productive Thoughts	Avoid Saying This	Why This Cues Unproductive Thoughts
	does not—deserve things based on perceptions of who has and has not tried hard enough. Inviting evaluations of deservingness gets in the way of the idea that everyone needs to have the support and resources they need to be healthy and well.		
People with high levels of sensitivity and thoughtfulness often experience greater distress when things do not feel like they are going well. But sensitivity and thoughtfulness are important and valuable attributes that predict a successful adulthood, with meaningful connections to others. Now is the time to learn to manage these skills so they benefit you the most and cause you the least distress.	This is strength-based framing. Importantly, it does not deny the distress but contextualizes it in existing strengths. Simultaneously, it states that part of development is learning to manage complex thoughts and feelings and that support can help the young person as they learn to do so.	You are too sensitive. –or– You think too much.	These messages are well intentioned but imply that feeling or thinking deeply is a problem rather than a source of strength when managed well. Further, these messages suggest an approach based on denying thoughts and feelings rather than learning to manage them.

Table 2
When speaking with a parent or caregiver about supporting their child

Say This	Why This Cues Productive Thoughts	Avoid Saying This	Why This Cues Unproductive Thoughts
Strong families cannot entirely prevent young people from experiencing challenges, but strong families can stand by children when they are experiencing distress and support them to get the professional guidance that can help.	Parents experience distress—and shame—when their children have an emotional, mental, or behavioral issue. This shame may prevent them from taking appropriate action. This message pushes back against the sense that they are failing and empowers families to know that their unwavering support *is* a vital action.	This is not your fault. Some adolescents just experience problems: That is just the way it is.	Leading with the word *fault* may backfire and activate the caregiver's feeling that it is actually, their fault. The second sentence reinforces the idea that adolescence is an inherently problematic phase, which normalizes inaction and "others" the young person.
Your child is experiencing a great deal of distress and would benefit from professional support. But you as the parent remain the most important person in their journey toward mental health. You may not be an expert on mental health, but you are the person who knows your child best. This is important and exactly what you need to be. You do not have to have all the answers; you just have to assure your child that no matter what, you will stand alongside them on this journey.	This statement provides the explicit information about what the parent should do by developing the idea of what it means to "stand by" an adolescent. This clear role and specific action can help dispel the crippling sense of doubt and inadequacy and empower parents.	Your child is experiencing mental health challenges and will benefit from professional support.	Although true, this statement does not give the parent a role to play. Furthermore, it may reinforce their sense of inadequacy for not being able to be their child's sole source of support. It leaves the door open for the parent's feelings of their own failure to take root.

(continued on next page)

Table 2
(continued)

Say This	Why This Cues Productive Thoughts	Avoid Saying This	Why This Cues Unproductive Thoughts
When one member of a family is experiencing mental, emotional, or behavioral challenges, the whole family experiences distress. That is why it is important that we work together to provide your family with the support that can help.	Many families feel badly that they cannot fix things when a child is distressed; they feel that they have failed. The framing here normalizes their own distress while inviting them to consider support that strengthens caregivers and attends to the needs of other siblings.	It is hard to have a child with a mental health condition.	This is an empathetic statement but is not solution focused and may reinforce a sense of helplessness and fatalism.
Adolescence is a time when children may experience very strong emotions. This is an important part of development and a sign that they are building their ability to read people, to empathize with others, and to navigate challenging interpersonal situations. These are all important social skills that we all need. Even though this is normal, they may need support to help them manage their rapidly developing emotional selves as they gain maturity.	This framing helps caregivers understand adolescent emotional development while conveying both the important and exciting aspects of emotional development with the need for adults to serve as active guides. Further, it gives an explanation about emotional development so that caregivers come away with a better understanding of this idea.	The emotional part of the adolescent brain develops sooner than the rational or reasoning part of the brain.	This common message cues the view of adolescents as highly emotional and without the capacity to reason. It powerfully "others" by framing the adolescent brain as fundamentally different, out of whack, and dysfunctional. It is a simple message that ignores the complexity of development; because it lacks explanation, it allows people to fill in their own view of what it means to be "emotional." Because of the cultural narrative about adolescents, people may fill this in as meaning "moody" or "irrational." In its most dangerous iteration, people will view irritability as "expected" rather than as a possible sign of depression. Finally, this simplistic message is too often interpreted as though adolescents lack rational thought altogether. This falsehood reinforces the idea that it is futile to help adolescents develop wise and protective thinking patterns.

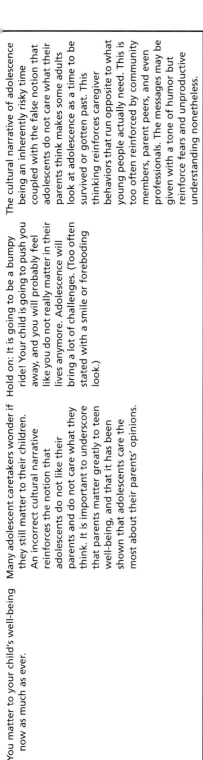

| You matter to your child's well-being now as much as ever. | Many adolescent caretakers wonder if they still matter to their children. An incorrect cultural narrative reinforces the notion that adolescents do not like their parents and do not care what they think. It is important to underscore that parents matter greatly to teen well-being, and that it has been shown that adolescents care the most about their parents' opinions. | Hold on: It is going to be a bumpy ride! Your child is going to push you away, and you will probably feel like you do not really matter in their lives anymore. Adolescence will bring a lot of challenges. (Too often stated with a smile or foreboding look.) | The cultural narrative of adolescence being an inherently risky time coupled with the false notion that adolescents do not care what their parents think makes some adults look at adolescence as a time to be survived or gotten past. This thinking reinforces caregiver behaviors that run opposite to what young people actually need. This is too often reinforced by community members, parent peers, and even professionals. The messages may be given with a tone of humor but reinforce fears and unproductive understanding nonetheless. |

Table 3
When speaking in a clinical setting about a potential problem or referring to further services

Say This	Why This Cues Productive Thoughts	Avoid Saying This	Why This Cues Unproductive Thoughts
Strong people seek support.	A common cultural narrative suggests that mental health is a weakness of character and that the need to seek service confirms an inability to individually handle problems. This framing flips that narrative and instead affirms help-seeking as a strength.	You need help.	This statement may cue the deficit model of mental and emotional health and reinforce feelings of shame or stigma about the help-seeking process.
Counseling and mental health services build on the strengths you already have.	This approach confirms that mental health services are not designed to change the participant but rather to access and build upon their existing strengths. This framing also avoids conveying a sense that adolescents are passive or powerless in addressing mental health challenges by clearly bringing their own skills and abilities into the conversation.	Counseling and mental health services will give you the answers you need to address your issue.	This approach reinforces a deficit model, suggesting that solutions come from the outside and do not involve the young person. It also falsely conveys the idea that there are nice and neat solutions ("answers") to mental health challenges, which creates misunderstanding.
Counseling and mental health services strengthen families.	This framing refutes the notion that mental and behavioral health systems replace families and pushes back on the idea that mental health challenges indicate family failure. It also advances the notion that active engagement can build skill sets in family systems.	Having a professional involved will take a lot of the weight off of your shoulders and lessen your worries about your child.	This approach cues the idea that services replace the role of caregivers. Although clearly designed to empathetically address parent concerns, it may generate resistance from an involved parent.

Many people experience mental and emotional distress. This means there are a lot of people who know what supports can help.	This framing normalizes the experience of distress. Many people may feel as though their suffering is unique and therefore they cannot be helped by professionals. This messaging reinforces the understanding that professionals are prepared and encourages help-seeking.	Kids in your generation are experiencing an unprecedented mental crisis, which means we need to work hard to find you a good therapist/counselor/psychiatrist.	This is a clear example of crisis messaging that reinforces helplessness and advances the idea that the problem is too big to really do anything about. This kind of message also reinforces the sense that there is a scarcity of "good" providers, which in turn may interfere with building a therapeutic alliance with existing services.
Mental health and emotional well-being are important aspects of overall health. Just like you would address a physical problem by seeking professional support, there are trained professionals who focus on this aspect of health.	Too many people who would access physical health care without shame view emotional, mental, or behavioral health as inherently shameful and therefore forego care. This messaging addresses this misunderstanding and integrates health care.	I am referring you to a professional to address your mental health.	There is nothing inherently wrong with this messaging. It is simple and clear. However, it misses the opportunity to integrate aspects of health care and minimize implicit shame or stigma.

Table 4
When speaking with a community audience about taking local action

Say This	Why This Cues Productive Thoughts	Avoid Saying This	Why This Cues Unproductive Thoughts
Adolescents are displaying both resilience and emotional distress in response to larger issues affecting our community and nation.	This approach ensures that adolescents are not portrayed in an overly simplistic or wholly negative way. It avoids blaming adolescents themselves for mental health challenges by painting a broader picture of responsibility and contextualizes adolescent distress as often reflecting societal problems, stressors, or inequities. It creates a sense that what surrounds us shapes and thereby offers a more complex—and accurate–image of adolescence today.	There is an adolescent mental health crisis.	Although it is true that many young people are experiencing distress, this message forgoes the opportunity to place the distress in a larger context, with a broader sense of responsibility that clearly extends beyond adolescents themselves. It could easily cue the understanding that adolescence is a highly vulnerable time and that adolescents are responsible for their own distress. Furthermore, the crisis message activates a sense of fatalism and advances the idea that this issue is too big to be addressed.
Adolescents are our future. For them to be prepared to lead us, we must provide the opportunities and support for them to develop their potential.	This framing reminds the community that investment in adolescents is a collective investment for the present and future.	The teens in this community are vulnerable. If they are going to make it, they need our support!	This frames adolescents as problematic and adults as fixing a problem rather than investing in youth as a solution. Furthermore, it "others" adolescents by labeling them as vulnerable and adopting an "us and them" positioning.
Adolescence is an amazing period of brain development. This development happens best in nurturing environments with engaged adults.	Many people do not know that the adolescent brain is actively shaped, and even fewer understand the role that adults, nurturing relationships, and supportive community environments play in this process.	The teen brain is very much a work in progress, which affects how young people act and behave.	Although this is an accurate statement, it advances a deficit perspective—that adolescent brains are somehow deficient. It also does nothing to position the critical role that adults and communities play in this process.

Adolescence is an opportunity to literally develop our future. We must enact strategies that contribute to positive youth development *and* give young people the added support to address their emotional mental or behavioral concerns.

Adolescence = opportunity. This bottom-line framing is needed to shift the cultural narrative. In the context of an uptick in mental health concerns, it reinforces that our goal is not the absence of distress but rather positive development. This message also stretches responsibility to include adults and society while not robbing adolescents of agency.

We must address mental health and emotional well-being.

Yes, but mental health needs to be contextualized in the overall goal of youth thriving and the framework of positive development or else we end up with partial and shortsighted solutions. Furthermore, the "we" here is a not a strong enough cue to counteract people's tendencies to see mental health as an issue of personal responsibility.

Table 5
When speaking with decision-makers about the need for policy and practice change

Say This	Why This Cues Productive Thoughts	Avoid Saying This	Why This Cues Unproductive Thoughts
Positive development happens in communities that are working to address equity issues so that all young people have what they need to develop to their potential.	It is critical to position equity as an essential, inseparable element of positive development. In equitable contexts, all youth flourish.	Your children and adolescents deserve more resources.	This framing may cue the notion that communities are competing over limited resources and that there is a zero-sum game. Too many communities believe that addressing equity means someone gains and does better while others lose and do worse. The word "your" in this framing may cue the scarcity model of thinking rather than the needed understanding that investment in positive development for *all* youth benefits everyone.
Strong families help young people become strong.	Strategies that support multiple generations support youth. These strategies are key to connect family well-being to adolescent well-being. For parents to effectively support young people, they need to have the supports to be healthy and empowered themselves. This messaging needs to be clear and consistent.	We must not ignore the needs of adolescents.	This framing ignores the connections between family and adolescent well-being and restricts the frame to include only young people. It cues the narrative that young people are the problem and puts the rest of society in the role of savior rather than partner.
There are youth who need focused attention and support, and we must ensure that there are adequate resources to address their mental, emotional, and behavioral needs and promote positive development.	This framing stands in contrast to many statements that label young people as "vulnerable" or "at risk" and inadvertently "other" and reinforce stigma and stereotypes. The statement also reinforces the	There is a youth mental health crisis, and we desperately need to create the resources needed for these vulnerable youth.	Speaking of a "crisis" may cue a mindset that resources are needed on a temporary basis but ultimately blocks the idea that real change is possible. This overarching statement also implies that

To effectively address the problems young people may be experiencing, we must engage the experts likely to give us the most actionable guidance—young people themselves.	sense that *positive* development is the goal, countering the overwhelming focus on crisis. The message also has a strong dose of collective responsibility to counter the default sense of individual responsibility for this issue. Finally, the message carefully avoids "deservingness" framing, which invites people to think about who really is deserving of support—and who is not. This locks thinking in an unproductive dynamic where people are evaluating individuals and groups to assess who *really* deserve public resources and social supports.	This framing creates a more expansive and accurate sense of expertise and avoids the idea that research or clinical knowledge is the only valid form of expertise. This framing boosts agency in young people and others, such as parents, who may be feel left out by framing that prioritizes research and clinical perspectives. It is essential that messages create space and advance framing that includes young people in active roles and positions them with power.
We must solve the problems youth are experiencing.	adolescence itself is a time of *storm and stress*. The term *vulnerable* is commonly used but undermines a young person by describing them in deficit terms. Instead, reframing this as "a youth placed at risk because of X circumstance" contextualizes the youth as navigating external forces or a challenging phase and puts responsibility on systems that must be changed rather than individuals who need to be fixed.	This framing creates a "savior/saved" dynamic in which young people (and parents) do not have power or agency in addressing challenges and are passive recipients rather than active agents in moving toward positive development and youth well-being.

reminding the young person that they can feel better, that they deserve to, and that you are there to support them, just as are those you may need to refer them to.[11] This framing counters fatalism, otherism, and individualism by promoting self-efficacy (there are things that can be done to make things better), a sense of a team, and the notion that the young person is of value.

To promote efficacy in mental well-being, note that there are things that can be done and that the young person plays a major role in these actions: Young people need to be active agents and play a role in the solutions we are advancing. This is an antidote to the feelings of fatalism and hopelessness that attach to this issue. This is relevant for youth who need additional support and youth trying to sustain optimal mental well-being. The use of "we" and "our" helps make it clear that young people are not alone in this or solely responsible for solutions. This approach counteracts individualism and the notion that solutions come only from individual effort, better choices, and drive. We also must make sure that young people receive the message that their needs are in addition to their own skills—a technique known as "additive framing." We may say we are offering "extra support" and providing support "in addition to the skills and strengths" that they already have. Instead of framing the young person as some incapable other, this positioning conveys the sense that the support builds on existing internal resources the young person already possesses. Using words such as *deserve* in a clinical setting can also remind youth that they have inherent strength, which is vital because people who have experienced shame need to know that they deserve attention.

Each of these strategies is tied to strength-based framing. Strength-based framing is about recognizing distress while always noting existing and potential future strengths. Strength-based framing positions development as a process of building skills on top of existing skills (skill begets skills) and getting better and better at managing complex thoughts and feelings.

When Speaking with a Parent or Caregiver About Supporting Their Child

Although youth can consent to their own care, if needed, it is important to remember that caregivers are vital members of the support team for a young person. In fact, youth often request pediatric professionals to help support improved communication with caregivers when they need additional supports. When that young person is struggling with mental illness, caregivers are more important than ever. Emphasizing this is a key strategy in strengthening the connection between caregivers and their teens by managing feelings of inefficacy that can activate fatalism. Pediatric professionals can be especially concrete about what the caregiver should do by developing the idea of what it means to "stand by" an adolescent. This clear sense of role, action, and agency can help dispel the sense of doubt and inadequacy that taps into fatalism and creates powerful and unproductive emotions in caregivers.

To effectively communicate with caregivers, pediatric professionals must also remember that parents experience distress—and shame—when their children have emotional, mental, or behavioral issues. This shame may prevent them from taking appropriate action. Overcoming that inaction can help a young person that is hesitant to engage caregivers gain confidence in the caregivers support role. Pediatric professionals' communications with parents must push back against the sense that parents are failing and instead make it clear that parents' unwavering support is among the most important things that can be done to address a mental health issue. Additionally, pediatric professionals must validate caregivers' own distress and the effect the young person's difficulties have on the family. This can be done explicitly while inviting caregivers to make sure their own emotional needs are met and that they are also attending to the needs of other siblings. In acknowledging these complex emotions and channeling them in more productive directions, this kind of messaging creates the sense that caregivers not only play a vital role but that they are not in it by themselves or solely responsible. This approach can help counter the sense of individualism and otherism with a more powerful sense of collective responsibility for the issue.

Further, pediatric caregivers should routinely reinforce to parents how much they matter in the lives of their adolescents. This conversation requires a shift from the false cultural narrative that says that not only is development on autopilot but adolescents reject adult guidance and care little what their parents say. We must lead with the truth: Parents are desired as guides for their adolescents, and young people care deeply about what their parents think and feel.[12,13]

When Speaking with Community Audiences and Decision-Makers About the Need for Change

In addition to the structural reframing noted earlier, better supporting adolescent mental well-being requires community and decision-maker engagement and action. Pediatric professionals are staunch advocates and effective advocacy for adolescents means avoiding narratives that activate the 3 mindsets discussed earlier. The goal is to cue more contextual, pragmatic, and collective thinking.

First, pediatric professionals need to ensure that adolescents are not portrayed in overly simplistic or wholly negative ways. This approach is key to avoiding the othering that much of the current narratives about adolescent mental health so powerfully fall into. Advocacy messages also need to advance solutions that highlight a broader picture of responsibility, countering senses of individualism that are attached to young people and caregivers and that prevent people from seeing the public and social nature of these issues. It needs to be clear that supporting positive adolescent development and well-being is a collective investment in the present and future. Contextualizing adolescent distress as often reflecting societal problems, stressors, or inequities creates a more complex—and accurate—image of adolescence.

It is also important to highlight the importance of promoting positive youth development and not just supporting adolescents in times of severe distress. Many people do not know that the adolescent brain is actively shaped, and even fewer understand the role that adults, especially supportive community environments, play in this process. Pediatric professionals need to work to shift the narrative from one that is problem and remedially focused to one that reinforces the goal of positive development (not merely the absence of distress).

Advocacy narratives must walk the line of creating a picture that includes adults and society but that does not rob adolescents of agency. Parents, caregivers, and community adults of many generations can and do provide meaningful support for youth. Family well-being and adolescent well-being are critically linked. For parents to support young people effectively, they need to have the support to be healthy and empowered themselves—a notion that must be clear and consistent in messaging. This framing has added value in that it can be used as a community strength–based message to show that community support that is already there can and should be used to promote well-being.

Community responsibility also means facing structural oppression as a root cause of mental distress. It is critical, therefore, to position equity as an essential, inseparable element of positive development and mental well-being. In equitable contexts, all youth flourish.

Importantly, pediatric professionals can and should discuss "deservingness" with individual young people in a clinical context because this can help validate an individual's right to care and healing. When speaking to communities and other stakeholders, pediatric professionals should avoid "deservingness" framing. In public advocacy, deservingness framing invites people to think about who *really* is deserving of support—and who is not. This framing cognitively creates an unproductive dynamic where people evaluate individuals and groups to assess who really deserves public resources and social supports and invites stereotypes and racist thinking that result in further marginalization of those who are already overburdened and underserved. Avoiding deservingness in this context means bypassing the negative pathways that some people may associate with "deserving" and instead focusing on solutions.

SUMMARY

Although the current narrative strives to address the mental health challenges faced by young people, it has negative unintended consequences that cannot be ignored. To truly support young people, we must reframe our communications and find a new narrative to share and tell. This narrative must emphasize agency and highlight the strengths and potential of young people and the common experiences that shape their well-being. It must move from a picture of "they" and "them" to one that makes it clear that supporting positive development and well-being is an "us" endeavor. The new narrative must have a place for young people, caregivers, health care professionals, the community, and broader society in the project of creating the conditions where *all* young people can be well and experience positive development. By understanding the mindsets that the current narrative activates and using the science of framing to find new strategies of positioning messages on this issue, we can shape a more supportive and productive discourse—one that gives young people what they need to be healthy and play an active role in their well-being.

DISCLOSURE

The authors have indicated they have no potential conflicts of interest to disclose.

REFERENCES

1. Holland D, Quinn N, editors. Cultural models in language and thought. Cambridge University Press; 1987.
2. Busso D, Volmert A, Kendall-Taylor N. Building opportunity into adolescence: mapping the gaps between expert and public understandings of adolescent development. Washington, DC: FrameWorks Institute; 2018.
3. Kendall-Taylor N. Shifting the frame to change how we see young people. J Adolesc Health 2020;66(2):137–9.
4. Busso DS, Pool AC, Kendall-Taylor N, et al. Reframing adolescent development: identifying communications challenges and opportunities. J Res Adolesc 2022; 32(4):1328–40.
5. Busso D, O'Neil M, Kendall-Taylor N. From risk to opportunity: framing adolescent development. Washington, DC: FrameWorks Institute; 2020.
6. Hall GS. Adolescence: its psychology and its relation to physiology, anthropology, sociology, sex, crime, religion, and education. New York, NY: D Appleton & Company; 1904.
7. Ginsburg KR, Pool AC, Brooks M, et al. Reframing adolescence: holding youth to high expectations and refuting undermining portrayals. In: Ginsburg KR, Ramirez McClain ZB, editors. Reaching teens: strength-based, trauma-sensitive, resilience-building communication strategies rooted in positive youth development.

2nd edition. Elk Grove Village, IL: American Academy of Pediatrics; 2020. p. 41–54.

8. Ginsburg KR. Focusing and building on existing strengths: a strategy to overcome risks and to prepare adolescents to be their best selves. In: Ginsburg KR, Ramirez McClain ZB, editors. Reaching teens: strength-based, trauma-sensitive, resilience-building communication strategies rooted in positive youth development. 2nd edition. Elk Grove Village, IL: American Academy of Pediatrics; 2020. p. 339–46.

9. Ginsburg KR, Rodriguez J. Reframing youth who have endured trauma and marginalization. In: Ginsburg KR, Ramirez McClain ZB, editors. Reaching teens: strength-based, trauma-sensitive, resilience-building communication strategies rooted in positive youth development. 2nd edition. Elk Grove Village, IL: American Academy of Pediatrics; 2020. p. 263–74.

10. Kendall-Taylor N, Ginsburg KR. Framing strategies to shape parent and adolescent understandings of development. Pediatrics 2021;148(3). https://doi.org/10.1542/peds.2021-050735. e2021050735.

11. Galinsky E. Ask the children: the breakthrough study that reveals how to succeed at work and parenting. New York, NY: Quill; 2000.

12. 5 Ways to #StandByTeens in support of teen mental health. Center for Parent and Teen Communication. 2023. Available at: https://parentandteen.com/support-teen-mental-health-stand-by-teens/. [Accessed 12 October 2023].

13. Ginsburg KR. The strength of seeking professional guidance. In: Ginsburg KR, editor. Congrats—you're having a teen!: strengthen your family and raise a good person. Elk Grove Village, IL: American Academy of Pediatrics; 2022. p. 315–24.

Mental Health, Climate Change, and Bodily Autonomy

An Analysis of Adolescent Health Policy in the Post-Pandemic Climate

Meredithe McNamara, MD, MSc[a],*, Jesse Barondeau, MD[b],
Joanna Brown, MD, MPH[c]

KEYWORDS

- Adolescents and young adults • Health policy • Social safety net
- Social determinants of health • Mental health • Climate change • Bodily autonomy

KEY POINTS

- The COVID-19 pandemic exacerbated the vulnerability of adolescents and young adults (AYAs) who face economic disadvantage, depend on social safety net resources, have politically targeted identities, are geopolitically displaced, and/or are racially/ethnically marginalized.
- A rapid change in social safety net policies has impacts that reverberate throughout inter-related domains of AYA health, especially for vulnerable AYAs.
- The authors analyze policy-related changes in mental health, climate change, and bodily autonomy to offer a paradigm for an equitable path forward.

INTRODUCTION

During the pandemic, disparities and biases in our society were thrown into high relief. Political extremism and conspiratorial thinking grew due to fatigue over COVID-19 safety measures.[1] Attitudes regarding science and medicine became more polarized, and mistrust of scientific authority became more common.[2] Regressive debate about gender, sexual orientation, reproductive health, and climate change ensued.[1,3] Among youth, financial insecurity, loneliness, and dependence on safety net resources during the pandemic were shown to predict medical mistrust.[4] Misinformation and

---

[a] Yale School of Medicine, 789 Howard Avenue, New Haven, CT 06519, USA; [b] University of Nebraska Medical Center, Children's Nebraska, 8200 Dodge Street, Omaha, NE 68114, USA; [c] Boston Children's Hospital, 333 Longwood Avenue, Boston, MA 02115, USA
* Corresponding author.
E-mail address: Meredithe.mcnamara@yale.edu

Pediatr Clin N Am 71 (2024) 729–744
https://doi.org/10.1016/j.pcl.2024.05.004   **pediatric.theclinics.com**

disinformation threatened essential aspects of public health such as infectious disease, climate change, sexual and reproductive health, and gender-affirming care.[2,5,6] Simultaneously, all levels of government demonstrated capability in crisis response. Communities collaborated to roll out home-based schooling, viral testing, and enhanced social programs. Expedited development and distribution of vaccines were a direct function of technological innovation and streamlined regulation.

These forces shaped a newer concept of vulnerability for adolescents and young adults (AYAs). The pandemic marked a time for many AYAs in which the weaknesses and resilience of their social safety nets were exposed. The social safety net refers to programs developed and supported through government policies, such as public insurance, food programs, unemployment support, education, and housing. We define vulnerable AYAs as people aged 11 to 25 years who face economic disadvantage, may depend on social safety net resources, have politically targeted identities, are geopolitically displaced, and/or are racially or ethnically marginalized (**Fig. 1**).

In declaring the end of the COVID-19 global health emergency, the World Health Organization Director-General Tedros Adhanom Ghebreyesus stated, "If we go back to how things were before… we will have failed to learn our lessons, and we will have failed future generations."[7] Moving forward, vulnerable AYAs stand to gain and lose a great deal. Our society has the tools to improve their health and well-being, but we are constrained by budgeting priorities and the sociopolitical environment. To illustrate these tensions, we discuss the pandemic-era catalysts and constraints to AYA health in 3 interrelated domains: mental health, climate change, and bodily autonomy (see **Fig. 1**). These areas are not comprehensive but do represent a broad perspective of adolescent life. Positive impacts on the lifespan follow when these areas receive proper investment and prioritization. We offer general guidance on a policy-focused path forward in these areas, informed by best available scientific evidence and health equity.

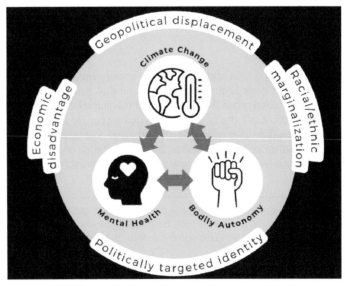

Fig. 1. Three interrelated aspects of adolescent and young adult health are shaped by pandemic-related forces that exacerbate AYA vulnerability.

THE SOCIAL SAFETY NET BEFORE, DURING, AND AFTER THE PANDEMIC

AYAs have long benefitted from interconnected policies that strengthen the social safety net and improve social determinants of health. Social determinants of health are the social, environmental, and economic conditions that influence well-being, some of which include socioeconomic status and access to health care, food, employment, and education. Governmental support of social safety net programs improved as COVID-19 intensified and fell as COVID-19 receded. Here, we review pandemic-related social safety net policies that shape social determinants of health for AYAs (**Table 1**).

Several policies supported access to health care and related services for AYAs prior to and during the pandemic. About 2.3 million young adults gained coverage from 2010 to 2013 due to the Affordable Care Act (ACA).[8] A higher income threshold for Medicaid qualification, optional by state, facilitated improved access to reproductive and preventive health services for AYAs, lesbian, gay, bisexual, transgender, and queer or questioning (LGBTQ+) people, and those in rural areas.[9] Insurers were required to offer coverage to young adults up to age 26 years on their parents' private insurance. The Children's Health Insurance Program remained open to children up to age 18 years for lower income families with incomes too high to qualify for Medicaid. During the pandemic, continuous Medicaid enrollment was instituted and about 23 million people gained coverage, about 7 million of whom were under age 19 years.[10] The Kaiser Family Foundation estimates that 8 to 24 million people will lose Medicaid as continuous enrollment stops and people must reapply and requalify.[10] Other federal and local programs supported AYA health prior to the pandemic and continue to do so. For instance, the Office of Population Affairs, in the Department of Health and Human Services (HHS), disburses teen pregnancy prevention funds and oversees the Title X family planning program, in which funds are disbursed to the states to provide free, confidential contraception. These offices may be focal points for future policy development for vulnerable AYAs.

Other pandemic-era policies temporarily strengthened social determinants of health such as economic stability, food access, and employment. The Supplemental Nutrition Assistance Program (SNAP) benefits provide food assistance to lower income families and individuals. The SNAP emergency allotments reduced the child poverty by about 14% in the last quarter of 2021, with most relief for Black and Hispanic/Latine people[11] but ended in March 2023. Expansion of the Child Tax Credit in 2021 also reduced the child poverty rate but expired with a predictable rebound in child poverty 1 year later.[12] From 2011 to 2017, scarcity of affordable housing worsened with a loss of 4 million units.[13] Emergency housing measures such as rental assistance and eviction moratoriums provided temporary relief at the height of the pandemic, but these programs were allowed to expire per a US Supreme Court ruling in 2021.[14]

MENTAL HEALTH AND WELL-BEING, CLIMATE CHANGE, AND BODILY AUTONOMY: AN INTERDEPENDENT PARADIGM

Pandemic-related forces that exacerbate AYA vulnerability, such as economic disadvantage, politically targeted identity, geopolitical displacement, and racial/ethnic marginalization, impede access to interrelated aspects of AYA health (see **Fig. 1**). To converge on the experiences of vulnerable AYAs, we discuss pandemic-related policies that impact mental health, climate change, and bodily autonomy. The mental health of vulnerable AYAs is inextricably tied to the stressors and challenges imposed by the climate crisis and policies that target bodily autonomy.[15,16] Concern over legal intrusion into personal health choices generates fear, anger, and sadness.[16] The

Table 1
A survey of some protective and harmful policies and actions impacting vulnerable adolescents and young adults and areas of need

		Protective Policies and Actions	Harmful Policies and Actions	Areas of Need
Social Safety Net	Insurance	Affordable Care Act Medicaid expansion before and during the pandemic Children's Health Insurance Program	*Braidwood v Becerra*, enjoined preventive care mandates of the Affordable Care Act	Maintenance of continuous Medicaid enrollment Medicaid enrollment across states to ensure universal AYA access to health insurance Reinstatement of pandemic-related assistance measures in the short term
	Antipoverty	Pandemic-related expansion of assistance measures: • Supplemental Nutrition Assistance Program emergency allotments • Child Tax Credit in 2021 • Eviction moratoriums, rental assistance	Expiration of pandemic-related assistance measures	
Mental Health	Access to care	Medicaid expansion Policies that allow telehealth and facilitate insurance reimbursement School-based mental health services • Enhanced funding of school-based health services (announced) • Department of Education proposal to eliminate parental consent for counseling services (not adopted) • States using American Rescue Act surplus funds for school-based services Introduction of 988 hotline	Conflicting and politicized anti-bodily autonomy priorities • Failure to pass Georgia Mental Health Parity Act at the expense of a state ban on gender-affirming care • Oklahoma state legislature stipulation disbursement of mental health funds is conditional upon cessation of gender-affirming medical care	Sustained Medicaid expansion
	Anti-racism	Cities and counties declaring racism as a public health crisis	Unraveling of the social safety net Weak hate crime legislation	Policies that address the toxicities of systemic and frame racism as a modifiable social determinant of health (eg, repair of the social safety net, federal anti-hate crime legislation)

Climate Change	Clean Air Act Paris Climate Agreement Inflation Reduction Act of 2022 Infrastructure Jobs and Investment Act The US city-based climate action plans State-based climate action lawsuits: *Held v Montana* (decision in favor of youth plaintiffs) Federal climate action lawsuit: *Juliana v United States* (pending trial)	Foreign and domestic policies contrary to environmental sustainability (eg, oil drilling in Alaska, geopolitical conflict)	Climate justice approach that prioritizes renewable energy, challenges disinformation
Bodily Autonomy Confidentiality	Title X	*Deanda v Becerra* State procurement of medical records of transgender patients	
HIV prevention	States that protect PrEP coverage	*Braidwood v Becerra* Tennessee refusal of federal HIV treatment and prevention funds	Federal legislation that codifies access to PrEP
Reproductive health	Shield laws that protect abortion Rulings that FDA approval of the first over-the-counter oral contraception pill	*Dobbs v Women's Health*, trigger bans and new legislation banning abortion *Alliance for Hippocratic Medicine v FDA*	Federal legislation that codifies equal protection for pregnancy-capable people
Attacks on LGBTQ+ rights	State shield laws that protect gender-affirming care Maine law that lowers age of consent of consent for gender-affirming care to 16 y	State laws banning gender-affirming care	Federal legislation that codifies equal protection for transgender and gender-diverse people

climate crisis denigrates bodily autonomy by forcing environmental harms on vulnerable AYAs and destabilizing their access to health care. This is not an exhaustive analysis, but may guide related efforts to understand how social policy and the pandemic impact areas in addition to mental health, climate change, and bodily autonomy.

Mental Health

Vulnerable AYAs were particularly susceptible to traumatic impacts of the pandemic. Many mental health issues worsened for all AYAs, including anxiety, attention deficit hyperactivity disorder (ADHD), substance use, and others.[17] The ability of AYAs to endure and recover from such challenges depends greatly on their interface with social determinants of health. Pandemic-era racism and minority stress amplified the suffering of vulnerable AYAs. Socioeconomic status impacted both risk of developing eating disorders and access to evidence-based care. Evolving pandemic-related policies impact the extent, quality, and delivery of a wide range of mental health services (see **Table 1**).

Worsening depressive symptoms were widely noted in AYAs,[17] but particularly concerning trends were noted among those who are racially or ethnically minoritized.[18] Scapegoating precipitated more racism and hate crimes toward Asian Americans. Asian American AYAs reported high rates of hypervigilance, verbal harassment, and threats.[19] Hostility toward Latine/Hispanic people grew in the United States, in tandem with pandemic-related border closures and politicized condemnation of migration from Central and South America.[20] As the homicides of George Floyd, Breonna Taylor, Ahmaud Arbery, and other Black Americans were widely covered in the media, Black AYAs experienced a growing awareness of racism and police brutality.[19] Many youth protested racial injustice and faced police brutality directly.[21,22] Lower income communities were heavily policed during lockdown measures and curfews.[23,24] Furthermore, death rates from COVID-19 infection were highest among Black, Latine/Hispanic, and Native American people.[25] AYAs were more likely to lose a caregiver and other members of their social networks.[26] The pandemic also led to increases in AYA suicide rates, disproportionately more among male individuals, those aged 5 to 12 and 18 to 24 years, and non-Hispanic American Indian, Alaskan Native, and Black youth.[27] Suicidal ideation and attempts also increased, with dramatic effects felt by pediatric intensive care units, emergency departments, and inpatient psychiatric services.[28] The 988 Lifeline, launched in 2022 after years of development, opens a new path for therapeutic, evidence-informed resources during crises, rather than police-driven responses.[29] Additional public education is needed to spread awareness of this service and enhance utilization. In 2020, 20 US cities and counties echoed medical consensus in declaring racism as a public health crisis.[30] It remains to be seen whether these designations drive much needed multisectoral, anti-racist policy change.

The pandemic-related increase and worsening severity of eating disorders were observed across all socioeconomic demographics, with some of the harshest effects felt among vulnerable AYAs.[31] Food insecurity, a risk factor for the development and worsening of eating disorders, disproportionately impacted economically vulnerable AYAs.[32] Nine states in the United States have no eating disorder treatment centers and there are very few certified family-based treatment specialists in the United States.[33] This long-standing underinvestment in eating disorder services and limited provider capacity to treat them became starkly obvious. Insurance reimbursement must be expanded for evidence-based eating disorder care and particularly for those with public insurance. Youth-serving clinicians need training to boost capacity.[33]

Expanded access of wraparound telehealth services for eating disorders is promising, and must widely accept Medicaid to serve the most vulnerable AYAs.[34–36]

Policies that impact mental health delivery in the social safety net for vulnerable AYAs are in flux. Increased admissions to treatment facilities and prescribing of commonly used psychiatric medications were noted during pandemic-related Medicaid expansion.[37] There have also been encouraging moves to fund and streamline mental health programming, particularly in the safety net setting of schools. In 2023, the HHS announced a large financial commitment to school-based mental health training and services, with a focus on substance use treatments.[38] The Department of Education proposed to eliminate parental consent prior to the receipt of counseling services to Medicaid billing in the Individuals with Disabilities Education Act.[39] (Several states already do not require parental consent for counseling services.) States, cities, and school systems have also directed surplus funds from the American Rescue Plan to enhance mental health programming.[40] However, conflicting policy priorities have derailed other attempts to improve services. The bipartisan Georgia Mental Health Parity Act of 2022 was intended to enforce compliance with federal mental health parity policy but expired before a vote at expense of an aggressive push to ban gender-affirming care for minors.[41] There are likely many other constructive policies that stalled or failed due to the anti-bodily autonomy political climate (see "Bodily Autonomy").

Climate Change

The climate crisis exerts concentrated harms on vulnerable AYAs during a pivotal period of life change. Weather emergencies overwhelm infrastructure and are linked to worsening health, including mental illness, respiratory and cardiac disease, environmental allergies, and infections such as Lyme, food insecurity, and adverse reproductive health outcomes.[42] Higher temperatures are linked to more emergency room visits for mental illness and higher suicide rates.[43,44] Racially and ethnically minoritized people in the United States are disproportionately harmed by the climate crisis.[45] The ecological environment is a social determinant of health that interacts with other determinants such as race/ethnicity, housing, and income.[46] An economically vulnerable person may, for instance, be more likely to reside in housing prone to flooding damage; climate-associated flooding would exacerbate their financial instability and likely harm their mental health. Ecoanxiety is a unique mental health consideration pertinent to the climate crisis. It is defined by the American Psychological Association as "the chronic fear of environmental cataclysm that comes from observing the seemingly irrevocable impact of climate change and the associated concern for one's future and that of next generations."[47] More than half of AYAs feel angry, anxious, and worried about climate change, but many also express feeling "motivated."[48,49] Increased engagement in climate activism is associated with improved well-being for AYAs experiencing ecoanxiety.[50]

Federal climate policies are welcome but insufficient thus far. The Environmental Protection Agency's Clean Air Act placed regulations on fossil fuel producers to reduce carbon emissions.[51] In 2015, the United States joined the Paris Climate Accords, a shared pledge of 196 countries to keep global warming below $2°C$.[52] (The United States pulled out of the accords in 2019 for politicized reasons and rejoined in 2021.[53]) Beginning 2 decades ago, US cities made "Climate Action Plans" (CAPs) and now, 45 large US cities have strong CAPs that represent 12% of the population.[54] In 2021, the Infrastructure Investment and Jobs Act was passed, which funded environmental protections, public health, and environmental justice initiatives for disadvantaged communities.[55] The Inflation Reduction Act in 2022 allocated the unprecedented amount of $386 billion for clean energy investment, tax incentives for electric vehicles, reduction of methane emissions, enhanced resiliency for communities that have borne the burden of climate change, and more.[56] At the same time, the United States continues to support policies contrary to sustainability and climate-related health progress, particularly regarding ongoing production of oil. In March 2023, the Biden administration approved drilling for oil off the Alaska coast.[57] The war in Ukraine and other global geopolitical events have had counterproductive effects on fossil fuel use and climate change as well.[58]

Youth activism presents innovative and impactful approaches to fostering policy-driven climate justice. In July 2023, a Montana judge ruled in favor of 16 youth who had sued the state for failing to protect their right to a clean environment.[59] These youth cited scientific evidence that burning fossil fuels contributes to global warming, which has adverse impacts on the plaintiffs' mental and physical health. The court affirmed that their "a fundamental constitutional right to a clean and healthful environment, which includes climate as part of the environmental life-support system." Several other similar youth-led cases are making their way through state courts. A national climate justice suit filed in 2016, *Juliana vs the United States*, involves a diverse cohort of 21 youth plaintiffs.[60] Many more grassroots and policy-level youth-led efforts are in play than can be covered in this piece.

A climate justice approach offers guidance for constructive policies moving forward. There are many frameworks for fostering climate justice, common themes of which include confronting disinformation and deepening our collective understanding of the interconnected forces that influence climate change, prioritizing the knowledge of indigenous peoples, showcasing the ways the people and places least responsible for climate change are most harmed by it, and prioritizing mitigation of climate-caused harms at the local level.

Bodily Autonomy

All AYAs in the post-pandemic era face legal intrusion into their bodily autonomy, with concentrated harms on vulnerable AYAs. Rising fear and mistrust of the medical establishment may have paved the way for some degree of public acceptance of legal measures that restrict standard medical care. Such legal measures include bans on abortion and gender-affirming care and judicial decisions that limit reproductive health, confidentiality, and preventive health care.

Clinical services that support AYA bodily autonomy are often offered under the same roof and are now targeted together. Community health centers, adolescent medicine clinics, and Planned Parenthood sites offer HIV prevention, gender-affirming care, and pregnancy options counseling. One way in which these comprehensive services face new threats is to their funding streams. Reauthorization of the Children's Hospital Graduate Medical Education Funding Act was amended in the US House of Representatives to defund pediatrics training programs in institutions that care for transgender youth (the fate of which is yet to be determined).[61] Oklahoma allocated $108 million in stimulus funds for mental health services, but on the condition that Oklahoma University Children's Hospital terminates clinical services for transgender youth.[62] These services are also the direct target of legal measures that criminalize their provision, such as in Nebraska, where abortion and gender-affirming care were banned in a single statute.[63] Additional attempts to restrict access to services include targeting insurance coverage and enacting decades-long statutes of limitations on malpractice lawsuits.[64] Many policies criminalize the provision of and consent to care and target those who "aid and abet" patients seeking care. Aiding and abetting can be legally construed as the act of transporting someone to receive medical services, providing child care for patients, and advising them on logistics, among others.[64] Many of the laws that arget aiding and abetting force extradition of patients who seek care outside their nome states. Demonstrating the regressive nature of such times, there have been no aws with extradition clauses in the United States since before the Civil War.[65]

Disinformation, as in many other areas of policy that impact or harm adolescent nealth, is used to justify legal intrusion into bodily autonomy. Disinformation describes the promulgation of information that is known to be false, with the intent to mislead. There are a few common ways in which disinformation may appear in policies that restrict bodily autonomy. Some actions are misinformed because they neglect key scientific truths. For example, Tennessee's refusal of Ryan White funds expressed a quiet denial of the state's HIV crisis, the effectiveness of prevention methods that had previously invested in, and a compelling government interest in protecting public health.[66] This move was widely recognized as a politically motivated attempt to exert control over community organizations that provide abortion services and gender-affirming care.[66] Likewise, *Dobbs vs Women's Health Organization* ended the constitutional right to abortion and demonstrated the Supreme Court's ignorance to the realities of human reproduction.[6] The harms of unsafe, unplanned, and undesired pregnancies are well-documented and yet the Court ruled in a way that neglected these truths completely. Some disinformation may be blatant and easily disproven but still influential. In 2020, an activist group called the Alliance for Hippocratic Medicine sued the Food and Drug Administration (FDA) to overturn mifepristone approval and made a series of false claims about the safety of the drug, including that it facilitates sex trafficking and often necessitates surgical abortion.[67] In 2023, FDA approval of mifepristone was overturned by a federal judge who relied on disinformation in his ruling, though an appeal is pending. Also, the Texas Attorney General claimed that prepubertal transgender children were routinely "sterilized" by physicians, thus justifying his 2022 legal opinion that the provision of gender-affirming care is child abuse.[68] Disinformation in legal measures that constrain bodily autonomy may be buried in layers of obfuscation. The misleading assertion that gender-affirming care is based on "low quality" evidence misuse technical terminology and neglect the fact that most medical care is informed by evidence derived from observational studies.[69] This claim, among others, has been used to justify bans on gender-affirming care for youth in 22 states thus far.[70]

Interference in confidentiality is another area where AYA bodily autonomy is at risk. In *Deanda v Becerra,* ruled against Title X confidentiality protections.[71] Arguing that Title X violates parents' "fundamental right to control and direct the upbringing of [their] children," this case presents one of the single greatest threats to AYA confidentiality in decades.[71] Over 176 federally funded clinics in Texas now must require parental consent for minors to receive contraception, with the potential to impact nationwide confidential access to services covered by Title X depending on how the case progresses through appeal. Other unprecedented threats to confidentiality include patient privacy violations driven by states themselves. Attorneys General in Missouri and Tennessee have demanded the records of patients receiving gender-affirming care and abortion services.[72,73] In Tennessee, 106 records containing patient identifiers of those receiving gender-affirming care were surrendered to the state Attorney General by Vanderbilt University Medical Center.[72]

Policy efforts to preserve AYA bodily autonomy have largely been reactive. Several states have enacted protections that preserve access to gender-affirming care and reproductive health, some in the same statutes.[74] Many of these laws also refuse compliance with aiding and abetting penalties elsewhere, although it is unlikely that such provisions protect recipients of care who return to home states where gender-affirming care or abortion are banned.[65] Maine passed a law that establishes the legal age of consent for gender-affirming care as 16 years, whereas by default it is 18 years in most other states.[75] The FDAs recent approval of the first over-the-counter oral contraceptive pill is a hopeful development that allows AYAs easier access to contraception and supports bodily autonomy, but cost may be a barrier.[76]

The outcomes of many state-based bans on reproductive health and gender-affirming care are in flux. Disinformation has been identified and criticized by judges in Arkansas, Florida, Alabama, Texas, Indiana, Kentucky, Tennessee, and Georgia, who ruled to enjoin or strike down bans on gender-affirming care. However, some injunctions have been overturned by higher courts, creating painful uncertainty for transgender youth and their families. There have been legal victories in reproductive health as well. A judge in Iowa enjoined the state's 6 week abortion ban, expressing sincere agreement with concerns about equal protections violations. These courts have also been receptive and deferential to the advocacy efforts of major medical organizations that have collaborated to submit amicus briefs in high profile cases.[77] As institutions make their own rules about what care they can provide, access to gender-affirming care and abortion services depends on more than just legal outcomes.

Researchers are working quickly to describe and quantify the harms of policies that restrict bodily autonomy. The 2023 *Braidwood v Beccera* decision, which struck down all preventive care mandates of the ACA and is on hold pending appeal, is predicted to cause over 2000 new HIV cases in the first year alone if cost sharing of pre-exposure prophylaxis (PrEP) for HIV fell by 10%.[78] Per new reports from the Centers for Disease Control (CDC), this would erase almost half of the gains made in prevention over the past few years.[79] (New infections fell from approximately 36,500 in 2017–32,100 in 2021, with the most dramatic improvements noted in AYAs.[79]) The Tennessee HIV funding reallocation is projected to cost $200 million in treatment of unprevented infections over 10 years.[66] The impact of a national abortion ban is projected to cause a 24% increase in maternal mortality across racial and ethnic groups, with a 39% increase anticipated for non-Hispanic Black people.[80] The American Association of Medical Colleges published data about worsening workforce shortages, showing that medical school graduates avoid matching into training programs in states with abortion bans.[81] Such research may educate policymakers and courts who seek to form protective, evidence-informed policies.

A PATH FORWARD THROUGH ADVOCACY

Advocacy for AYAs in the post-pandemic climate must be informed an unflinching examination of how COVID-19 exacerbated their vulnerability. Pediatricians should assess their own strengths as assets in the support and protection of vulnerable AYAs. Such strengths may include public speaking, media engagement, research, networking, grassroots partnership, and the amplification of youth voices. Analyzing the intersection of mental health, climate change, and bodily autonomy reveals strategic courses that can protect vulnerable AYAs moving forward.

First, financial sustenance of social safety net programs must be secured because future emergencies are inevitable. This is particularly urgent as many programs face paradoxic post-pandemic rollbacks. Inattention to the benefits of pandemic-era social safety net expansion is setting in, and this should be challenged. Pediatricians should call for sustenance of pandemic-era social safety net expansion. The vulnerabilities caused and exacerbated by COVID-19 are complex, intertwined, and likely to persist long after the end of the global health emergency. The weaknesses in the social safety net revealed by COVID-19 should be viewed as opportunities for constructive and innovative policy.

Second, we face a new, dire need for integrity standards in health policy. Disinformation has been successfully weaponized because there are no safeguards to prevent the misrepresentation of fact in law. The involvement of health advocates, clinical experts, and youth in legal processes must continue–despite and because of the harsh political climate they face. Medical societies may consider proactively issuing such integrity standards to supply policymakers with true information about health conditions impacted by policy, standard medical practices, the safety of evidence that informs care being regulated.

Third, youth-serving clinicians and scholars must practice clinical care and conduct research informed by pandemic-related concepts regarding the social determinants of health. As we advocate for and await sustainable policy solutions, we must identify and address the systematic effects of disinformation, racism, and resource deprivation in the interrelated aspects of AYA health. Our patients need their health care and the policies that affect access to that care to be grounded in the realities and new vulnerabilities they face.

CLINICS CARE POINTS

- Providers who serve AYAs should consider features of the post-pandemic climate that make AYAs particularly vulnerable.
- Providers who serve AYAs have a newly important role to play in advocating for social safety net programs and evidence-based policy that supports the well-being of their patients.

DISCLOSURE

The authors have nothing to disclose.

REFERENCES

1. Jorgensen F, Bor A, Rasmussen MS, et al. Pandemic fatigue fueled political discontent during the COVID-19 pandemic. Proc Natl Acad Sci U S A Nov 29 2022;119(48). https://doi.org/10.1073/pnas.2201266119. e2201266119.
2. Perlis RH, Lunz Trujillo K, Green J, et al. Misinformation, Trust, and Use of Ivermectin and Hydroxychloroquine for COVID-19. JAMA Health Forum 2023;4(9): e233257. https://doi.org/10.1001/jamahealthforum.2023.3257.
3. Hotez PJ. Anti-science extremism in America: escalating and globalizing. Microbes Infect Nov-Dec 2020;22(10):505–7. https://doi.org/10.1016/j.micinf.2020.09.005.
4. Ash MJ, Berkley-Patton J, Christensen K, et al. Predictors of medical mistrust among urban youth of color during the COVID-19 pandemic. Transl Behav Med 2021;11(8):1626–34. https://doi.org/10.1093/tbm/ibab061.
5. McNamara M, Lepore C, Alstott A. Protecting Transgender Health and Challenging Science Denialism in Policy. N Engl J Med 2022;387(21):1919–21. https://doi.org/10.1056/NEJMp2213085.
6. Lawmakers v. The Scientific Realities of Human Reproduction. N Engl J Med 2022. https://doi.org/10.1056/NEJMe2208288.
7. World Health Organization. WHO Director-General opening remarks at the media briefing - 5 May 2023. Available at: https://www.who.int/news-room/speeches/item/who-director-general-s-opening-remarks-at-the-media-briefing—5-may-2023. [Accessed 1 October 2023].

8. Health Affairs. Record high ACA enrollment at 31 million Americans. Available at: https://www.healthaffairs.org/content/forefront/record-high-aca-enrollment-31-million-americans. [Accessed 1 October 2023].

9. Darney BG, Jacob RL, Hoopes M, et al. Evaluation of Medicaid Expansion Under the Affordable Care Act and Contraceptive Care in US Community Health Centers. JAMA Netw Open 2020;3(6):e206874. https://doi.org/10.1001/jamanetworkopen.2020.6874.

10. Tolbert J. 10 things to know about the unwinding of the Medicaid continuous enrollment provision. Kaiser Family Foundation. Available at: https://www.kff.org/medicaid/issue-brief/10-things-to-know-about-the-unwinding-of-the-medicaid-continuous-enrollment-provision/. [Accessed 1 October 2023].

11. Rosenbaum DBK, Hall L. Temporary Pandemic SNAP Benefits Will End in Remaining 35 States in March 2023. Center on Budget and Policy Priorities. Available at: https://www.cbpp.org/research/food-assistance/temporary-pandemic-snap-benefits-will-end-in-remaining-35-states-in-march. [Accessed 1 October 2023].

12. Institute on Taxation and Economic Policy. Lapse of Expanded Child Tax Credit Led to Unprecedented Rise in Child Poverty. Available at: https://itep.org/lapse-of-expanded-child-tax-credit-led-to-unprecedented-rise-in-child-poverty-2023/. [Accessed 1 October 2023].

13. Benfer EA, Vlahov D, Long MY, et al. Eviction, Health Inequity, and the Spread of COVID-19: Housing Policy as a Primary Pandemic Mitigation Strategy. J Urban Health 2021;98(1):1–12. https://doi.org/10.1007/s11524-020-00502-1.

14. Alabama Association of Realtors, Department of Health and Human Services, In: Supreme court of the United States. 2021.

15. van Nieuwenhuizen A, Hudson K, Chen X, et al. The Effects of Climate Change on Child and Adolescent Mental Health: Clinical Considerations. Curr Psychiatr Rep 2021;23(12):88. https://doi.org/10.1007/s11920-021-01296-y.

16. Allison BA, Vear K, Hoopes AJ, et al. Adolescent Awareness of the Changing Legal Landscape of Abortion in the United States and Its Implications. J Adolesc Health 2023;73(2):230–6. https://doi.org/10.1016/j.jadohealth.2023.04.008.

17. Liu SR, Davis EP, Palma AM, et al. The acute and persisting impact of COVID-19 on trajectories of adolescent depression: Sex differences and social connectedness. J Affect Disord 2022;299:246–55. https://doi.org/10.1016/j.jad.2021.11.030.

18. Liu SR, Davis EP, Palma AM, et al. Experiences of COVID-19-Related Racism and Impact on Depression Trajectories Among Racially/Ethnically Minoritized Adolescents. J Adolesc Health 2023;72(6):885–91. https://doi.org/10.1016/j.jadohealth.2022.12.020.

19. Chae DH, Yip T, Martz CD, et al. Vicarious Racism and Vigilance During the COVID-19 Pandemic: Mental Health Implications Among Asian and Black Americans. Publ Health Rep Jul-Aug 2021;136(4):508–17. https://doi.org/10.1177/00333549211018675.

20. Foxen P. Latinos C, and social belonging: voices from the community. UnidosUS; 2021.

21. Kaske EA, Cramer SW, Pena Pino I, et al. Injuries from Less-Lethal Weapons during the George Floyd Protests in Minneapolis. N Engl J Med 2021;384(8):774–5. https://doi.org/10.1056/NEJMc2032052.

22. Chaudhary MJ, Richardson J Jr. Violence Against Black Lives Matter Protestors: a Review. Curr Trauma Rep 2022;8(3):96–104. https://doi.org/10.1007/s40719-022-00228-2.

23. Jahn JL, Simes JT, Cowger TL, et al. Racial Disparities in Neighborhood Arrest Rates during the COVID-19 Pandemic. J Urban Health 2022;99(1):67–76. https://doi.org/10.1007/s11524-021-00598-z.

24. Kajeepeta S, Bruzelius E, Ho JZ, et al. Policing the pandemic: Estimating spatial and racialized inequities in New York City police enforcement of COVID-19 mandates. Crit Publ Health 2022;32(1):56–67. https://doi.org/10.1080/09581596.2021.1987387.

25. Ahmad FB, Cisewski JA, Xu J, et al. COVID-19 Mortality Update - United States, 2022. MMWR Morb Mortal Wkly Rep 2023;72(18):493–6. https://doi.org/10.15585/mmwr.mm7218a4.

26. Hillis SD, Blenkinsop A, Villaveces A, et al. COVID-19-Associated Orphanhood and Caregiver Death in the United States. Pediatrics 2021;148(6). https://doi.org/10.1542/peds.2021-053760.

27. Bridge JA, Ruch DA, Sheftall AH, et al. Youth Suicide During the First Year of the COVID-19 Pandemic. Pediatrics 2023;151(3). https://doi.org/10.1542/peds.2022-058375.

28. Hill RM, Rufino K, Kurian S, et al. Suicide Ideation and Attempts in a Pediatric Emergency Department Before and During COVID-19. Pediatrics 2021;147(3). https://doi.org/10.1542/peds.2020-029280.

29. Suran M. How the New 988 Lifeline Is Helping Millions in Mental Health Crisis. JAMA 2023;330(11):1025–8. https://doi.org/10.1001/jama.2023.14440.

30. Vestal C. Racism is a public health crisis, say cities and counties. Pew Stateline. Available at: https://www.pewtrusts.org/en/research-and-analysis/blogs/stateline/2020/06/15/racism-is-a-public-health-crisis-say-cities-and-counties. [Accessed 1 October 2023].

31. Gilsbach S, Plana MT, Castro-Fornieles J, et al. Increase in admission rates and symptom severity of childhood and adolescent anorexia nervosa in Europe during the COVID-19 pandemic: data from specialized eating disorder units in different European countries. Child Adolesc Psychiatr Ment Health 2022;16(1):46. https://doi.org/10.1186/s13034-022-00482-x.

32. Urban B, Jones N, Freestone D, et al. Food insecurity among youth seeking eating disorder treatment. Eat Behav 2023;49:101738. https://doi.org/10.1016/j.eatbeh.2023.101738.

33. Lebow J, O'Brien JRG, Mattke A, et al. A primary care modification of family-based treatment for adolescent restrictive eating disorders. Eat Disord Jul-Aug 2021;29(4):376–89. https://doi.org/10.1080/10640266.2019.1656468.

34. Steinberg D, Perry T, Freestone D, et al. Effectiveness of delivering evidence-based eating disorder treatment via telemedicine for children, adolescents, and youth. Eat Disord Jan-Feb 2023;31(1):85–101. https://doi.org/10.1080/10640266.2022.2076334.

35. Wood SM, White K, Peebles R, et al. Outcomes of a Rapid Adolescent Telehealth Scale-Up During the COVID-19 Pandemic. J Adolesc Health 2020;67(2):172–8. https://doi.org/10.1016/j.jadohealth.2020.05.025.

36. North S. Expanding Telehealth in Adolescent Care: Moving Beyond the COVID-19 Pandemic. Pediatrics 2023;151(Suppl 1). https://doi.org/10.1542/peds.2022-057267J.

37. Ortega A. Medicaid Expansion and mental health treatment: Evidence from the Affordable Care Act. Health Econ 2023;32(4):755–806. https://doi.org/10.1002/hec.4633.

38. Substance Use and Mental Health Administration. The Biden-Harris Administration Awards More Than $88 Million in Grants that Safeguard Youth Mental Health and Expand Access to Treatment for Substance Use Disorders. Available at: https://www.samhsa.gov/newsroom/press-announcements/20230811/biden-harris-admi nistration-awards-grants-safeguard-youth-mental-health-expand-access-treatme nt-substance-use-disorders#:~:text=The%20grant%20programs%20serve%20- a,use%20disorder%20(SUD)%20treatments. [Accessed 1 October 2023].

39. Federal Register. Assistance to States for the Education of Children With Disabilities. Available at: https://www.federalregister.gov/documents/2023/05/18/2023-10542/ assistance-to-states-for-the-education-of-children-with-disabilities. [Accessed 1 October 2023].

40. Vestal C. Awash in Federal Money, State Lawmakers Tackle Worsening Youth Mental Health. Stateline. Available at: https://stateline.org/2023/03/17/awash-in-federal-mon ey-state-lawmakers-tackle-worsening-youth-mental-health/. [Accessed 1 October 2023].

41. Eldridge E, Gratas S. A bill to increase funding for mental health failed to pass the Senate. What happened, what's next. Georgia Public Broadcasting. Available at: https://www.gpb.org/news/2023/03/31/bill-increase-funding-for-mental-health- failed-pass-the-senate-what-happened-whats. [Accessed 1 October 2023].

42. Health Ca. Centers for Disease Control. Available at: https://www.cdc.gov/cli- mateandhealth/effects/default.htm. [Accessed 1 October 2023].

43. Sun S, Weinberger KR, Nori-Sarma A, et al. Ambient heat and risks of emergency department visits among adults in the United States: time stratified case cross- over study. BMJ 2021;375:e065653. https://doi.org/10.1136/bmj-2021-065653.

44. Dring P, Armstrong M, Alexander R, et al. Emergency Department Visits for Heat- Related Emergency Conditions in the United States from 2008-2020. Int J Environ Res Publ Health 2022;19(22). https://doi.org/10.3390/ijerph192214781.

45. Berberian AG, Gonzalez DJX, Cushing LJ. Racial Disparities in Climate Change- Related Health Effects in the United States. Curr Environ Health Rep 2022;9(3): 451–64. https://doi.org/10.1007/s40572-022-00360-w.

46. World Meteorological Association. Global temperatures set to reach new records in next five years. Available at: https://public.wmo.int/en/media/press-release/global- temperatures-set-reach-new-records-next-five-years. [Accessed 1 October 2023].

47. Clayton S, Manning CM, Krygsman K, et al. Mental health and our changing climate: impacts, implications, and guidance. Washington, D.C.: American Psy- chological Association, and ECOAMERICA; 2017.

48. Hamel L, Lopes L, Muñana C, et al. The Kaiser Family Foundation/Washington Post Climate Change Survey. Available at: https://www.kff.org/other/report/the- kaiser-family-foundation-washington-post-climate-change-survey/. [Accessed 1 October 2023].

49. Clemens V, von Hirschhausen E, Fegert JM. Report of the intergovernmental panel on climate change: implications for the mental health policy of children and adolescents in Europe-a scoping review. Eur Child Adolesc Psychiatr 2022;31(5):701–13. https://doi.org/10.1007/s00787-020-01615-3.

50. Ojala M, Bengtsson H. Young People's Coping Strategies Concerning Climate Change: Relations to Perceived Communication With Parents and Friends and Proenvironmental Behavior. Environ Behav 2018;51(8):907–35. https://doi.org/ 10.1177/0013916518763894.

51. Environmental Protection Agency. Overview of the Clean Air Act and air pollution. Available at: https://www.epa.gov/clean-air-act-overview. [Accessed 1 October 2023].
52. United Nations. The Paris Climate Agreement. Available at: https://unfccc.int/process-and-meetings/the-paris-agreement. [Accessed 1 October 2023].
53. National Public Radio. U.S. officially leaving Paris climate agreement. Available at: https://www.npr.org/2020/11/03/930312701/u-s-officially-leaving-paris-climate-agreement. [Accessed 1 October 2023].
54. Markolf SAI, Muro M, Victor D. Pledges and progress: steps toward greenhouse gas emissions reductions in the 100 largest cities across the United States. The Brookings Institute. Available at: https://www.brookings.edu/articles/pledges-and-progress-steps-toward-greenhouse-gas-emissions-reductions-in-the-100-largest-cities-across-the-united-states/. [Accessed 1 October 2023].
55. The White House. The bipartisan infrastructure deal boosts clean energy jobs, strengthens resilience and advances environmental justice. Available at: https://www.whitehouse.gov/briefing-room/statements-releases/2021/11/08/fact-sheet-the-bipartisan-infrastructure-deal-boosts-clean-energy-jobs-strengthens-resilience-and-advances-environmental-justice/. [Accessed 1 October 2023].
56. CNBC. The U.S. passed a historic climate deal this year – here's a recap of what's in the bill. Available at: https://www.cnbc.com/2022/12/30/2022-climate-recap-whats-in-the-historic-inflation-reduction-act.html. [Accessed 1 October 2023].
57. Friedman LKrauss C. Pristine Alaska, an oil giant prepares to drill for decades. Available at: https://www.nytimes.com/2023/04/06/climate/willow-alaska-oil-biden.html. [Accessed 1 October 2023].
58. Gelles D. The War in Ukraine Upended Energy Markets. What Does That Mean for the Climate? The New York Times. Available at: https://www.nytimes.com/2023/01/14/business/energy-environment/davos-energy-climate-ukraine.html. [Accessed 1 October 2023].
59. ABC News. Montana youths win lawsuit against state for failing to protect them against fossil fuels. Available at: https://abcnews.go.com/US/montana-youths-win-climate-lawsuit-fossil-fuels/story?id=102260674. [Accessed 1 October 2023].
60. Our Children's Trust. Juliana v United States. Available at: https://www.ourchildrenstrust.org/court-orders-and-pleadings. [Accessed 1 October 2023].
61. Goldman M. Pediatric training funds ensnared in trans care debate. Axios. Available at: https://www.axios.com/2023/06/28/pediatric-training-trans-care-debate. [Accessed 1 October 2023].
62. Forman C. Stitt signs bill blocking some gender care for transgender youth at OU Children's Hospital. The Oklahoman. Available at: https://www.oklahoman.com/story/news/politics/2022/10/04/oklahoma-governor-kevin-stitt-blocks-ou-childrens-hospital-gender-affirming-care/69538239007/. [Accessed 1 October 2023].
63. Let Them Grow and Preborn Child Protection Act. 2023. Available at: https://nebraskalegislature.gov/bills/view_bill.php?DocumentID=49961. [Accessed 1 October 2023].
64. Mallory C, Chin MG, Lee JC. Legal Penalties for Physicians Providing Gender-Affirming Care. JAMA 2023;329(21):1821–2. https://doi.org/10.1001/jama.2023.8232.
65. Caraballo A, Conti-Cook C, Pierre Y, et al. Extradition in Post-Roe America. The City University of New York Law Review 2023;26(1).
66. Tran NM, Rebeiro P, McKay T. Tennessee Rejects Federal HIV Prevention Funds: A Looming Public Health And Financial Disaster. Health Affairs Forefront 2023.

67. Zettler PJ, Adashi EY, Cohen IG. Alliance for Hippocratic Medicine v. FDA - Dobbs's Collateral Consequences for Pharmaceutical Regulation. N Engl J Med 2023;388(10):e29. https://doi.org/10.1056/NEJMp2301813.
68. Boulware S, Kamody R, Kuper L, et al. Biased science: the Texas and Alabama measures criminalizing medical treatment for transgender children and adolescents rely on inaccurate and misleading scientific claims. Yale University. Available at: https://medicine.yale.edu/lgbtqi/research/gender-affirming-care/report%20on%20the%20science%20of%20gender-affirming%20care%20final%20april%2028%202022_442952_55174_v1.pdf. [Accessed 1 October 2023].
69. Fleming PS, Koletsi D, Ioannidis JP, et al. High quality of the evidence for medical and other health-related interventions was uncommon in Cochrane systematic reviews. J Clin Epidemiol 2016;78:34–42. https://doi.org/10.1016/j.jclinepi.2016.03.012.
70. Human Rights Campaign. Map: attacks on gender affirming care by state. Available at: https://www.hrc.org/resources/attacks-on-gender-affirming-care-by-state-map. [Accessed 1 October 2023].
71. Deanda v. Becerra N-c–Z, slip op. at p.51 (N.D. Tex. 2022).
72. Mattisse J. Transgender patients sue the hospital that provided their records to Tennessee's attorney general. Associated Press. Available at: https://apnews.com/article/tennessee-transgender-patient-records-vanderbilt-f188c6c0c97145-75554867b4541141dd. [Accessed 1 October 2023].
73. Hospital sues Missouri's top prosecutor over trans care data. Associated Press. Available at: https://apnews.com/article/transgender-care-missouri-attorney-general-hospital-lawsuit-217e78b46cfd50432c97e3cc759f9717. [Accessed 1 October 2023].
74. Movement Advancement Project. Transgender health "shield" laws. Available at: https://www.lgbtmap.org/equality-maps/healthcare/trans_shield_laws#: ~ :text= These%20"shield"%20or%20"refuge,to%20transgender%2Drelated%20health%20care. [Accessed 1 October 2023].
75. Maine House votes to ensure teens can receive gender-affirming health care. Associated Press. Available at: https://apnews.com/article/maine-gender-affirming-care-8cfe628978535b1833c023256643a5f1. [Accessed 1 October 2023].
76. Tanne JH. FDA approves daily over-the-counter oral contraceptive with no age restrictions. BMJ 2023;382:p1631. https://doi.org/10.1136/bmj.p1631.
77. Brief of Amicus Curiae American Academy of Pediatrics and Additional National and State Medical and Mental Health Organizations in Support of Plaintiffs' Motion for Temporary Restraining Order and Preliminary Injunction. Eknes-Tucker v. Ivey [later renamed Eknes-Tucker v. Abbott] 2022.
78. Paltiel AD, Ahmed AR, Jin EY, et al. Increased HIV Transmissions With Reduced Insurance Coverage for HIV Preexposure Prophylaxis: Potential Consequences of Braidwood Management v. Becerra. Open Forum Infect Dis 2023;10(3): ofad139. https://doi.org/10.1093/ofid/ofad139.
79. Center for Disease Control. Available at: https://www.cdc.gov/media/releases/2023/p0523-hiv-declines-among-young-people.html. [Accessed 1 October 2023].
80. Stevenson A Root L, Menken J. The maternal mortality consequences of losing abortion access 2022. https://doi.org/10.31235/osf.io/7g29k.
81. Orgera K, Mahmood H, Grover A. Training location preferences of U.S. Medical school graduates post Dobbs v. Jackson Women's Health Organization Decision; 2023. https://doi.org/10.15766/rai_2rw8fvba.

Anti-racism, Heterosexism, and Transphobia

Strategies for Adolescent Health Promotion Post-Coronavirus Disease 2019

Dia Binitie Thurston, PhD[a,b,*], Rebecca L. Fix, PhD[c],
Elizabeth Getzoff Testa, PhD[d]

KEYWORDS

- Disparity • Sexual orientation • Youth • Equity • Gender identity • Race
- Anti-black racism

KEY POINTS

- Adolescent health practitioners and researchers require an intersectional lens in order to provide culturally responsive care, yet current educational and training curriculum do not center intersectional perspectives.
- The role of intersectionality in driving health inequities has also been under examined.
- The authors present the Self-examination, Talk, Yield time and space to learn from youth, Learn about intersectionality and health inequity, Evaluate policies and practices (STYLE) framework, adapted to address health inequity.
- The health-equity adapted STYLE framework can be used by adolescent health experts to counter their own biases and actively address anti-Black racism, heterosexism, and transphobia within clinical and research encounters.

INTRODUCTION

Anti-Black Racism, heterosexism, and transphobia are significant public health concerns that contribute to poor adolescent health. Within adolescent health care settings, such discrimination impacts health outcomes in the short and long term. Many

[a] Department of Health Sciences and Applied Psychology, Northeastern University, 360 Huntington Avenue, Boston, MA 02115, USA; [b] Institute for Health Equity and Social Justice Research, Northeastern University, 360 Huntington Avenue, 322 INV, Boston, MA 02115, USA; [c] Department of Mental Health, Johns Hopkins Bloomberg School of Public Health, 415 North Washington Street Room 519, Baltimore, MD 21231, USA; [d] Department of Psychology and Neuropsychology, Mt Washington Pediatric Hospital, 1708 West Rogers Avenue, Baltimore, MD 21209, USA
* Corresponding author. Department of Applied Psychology, Institute for Health Equity and Social Justice, Northeastern University, 360 Huntington Avenue, 322 INV, Boston, MA 02115.
E-mail address: i.thurston@northeastern.edu

Pediatr Clin N Am 71 (2024) 745–760
https://doi.org/10.1016/j.pcl.2024.04.008
0031-3955/24/© 2024 Elsevier Inc. All rights reserved.

pediatric.theclinics.com

professionals working in adolescent health, pediatric psychology, and pediatric care settings are ill-equipped to serve youth with marginalized and oppressed identities due to limited focus on these populations in their training and educational curriculum. In the current discourse, the authors provide a brief overview of anti-Black racism, heterosexism, transphobia; associated intersectional discrimination; and impact on adolescent health inequities. The authors introduce the health-equity adapted Self-examination, Talk, Yield time and space to learn from youth, Learn about intersectionality and health inequity, Evaluate policies and practices (STYLE) framework and use case examples to demonstrate how STYLE strategies can be applied to promote adolescent health post-coronavirus disease 2019 (COVID-19).

Anti-Black Racism and Its Role in Health Care

There are significant disparities in life expectancy and health outcomes in the United States, such that on average, Black adults have a substantially lower life expectancy and worse health outcomes relative to White adults.[1] Social determinants/drivers of health inequities, include factors such as limited access to quality food, housing segregation, and disproportionate burden of debt (**Box 1**). Collectively, social factors initiate, drive, and maintain health inequities in populations made vulnerable by structural discrimination.[2,3] Anti-Black racism (hence forth referred to as racism; see **Box 1**) is a well-established social driver/determinant of health in the United States[4] and beyond.[5] A structural definition of racism is one that labels racism as a sociopolitical, White supremacist system that categorizes social groups of people using a hierarchical model into races for the primary purpose of inequitable allocation of power, resources, and status.[6] The medical educational curriculum is steeped in White supremacy and anti-Black racism due to lack of diverse medical faculty, limited teaching on the history of White supremacy and how it maintains teaching of racist tropes, corporatization of medicine, and much more.[7] The racialized social system plays out in other systems beyond education, including health care and permeates interactions with the health care system from access to utilization and all points between.[3]

Health Consequences of Anti-Black Racism Among Adolescents in Pediatric Care Settings

Black youth are disproportionately exposed to different forms of structural anti-Black racism including racist miseducation, racist dis/misinformation, online racial discrimination and race-based trauma, racist privacy violations and surveillance, and racist health/health care algorithms and tech processes.[8] These forms of structural racism impact various sectors of adolescent health care including provider bias/discrimination, health leadership bias/discrimination, and health care coverage, all of which ultimately drive racial health disparities in medical morbidity and mortality.[8] Due to

---

Box 1
Key terminology

Social Determinants/Drivers of Health Inequities: framework that classifies social interactions (such as limited quality food access, housing segregation, disproportionate, burden of debt, etc.) together as maintaining health inequities in populations made vulnerable by structural discrimination.

Structural Anti-Black Racism: labels racism as a sociopolitical, White supremacist system that categorizes social groups of people using a hierarchical model into races for the primary purpose of inequitable allocation of power, resources, and status.

structural anti-Black racism, Black youth are also disproportionately exposed to community violence,[9] social drivers/determinants of health,[10] and toxic stress[11] which further decrease their likelihood of obtaining appropriate, tailored, and responsive care in pediatric health care settings, and which ultimately drive health inequities. Health consequences of anti-Black racism span a broad range. For example, a recent study showcased systemic contributions to the disparate rates of psychiatric illness in Black and White children due to Black youth having disproportional childhood exposure to material hardship and traumatic events which in turn are linked to lower amygdala, hippocampus, and prefrontal context gray matter volume compared to White youth.[11] Other researchers have shown how racism is linked to lower mental health utilization and reduced intervention efficacy even when services are utilized.[12,13]

Resilience and Protective Factors Against Anti-Black Racism

Amid long-standing anti-Black racism, Black youth also embody resilience, have protective factors, and showcase a variety of lived experiences that highlight the heterogeneity of their experiences. In this article, the authors emphasize the importance of advancing the under-discussed strengths of Black youth and they suggest ways to ensure that adolescent health providers support these youth as whole people rather than advancing a "single story"[14] of Black youth experiences. Adolescent health professionals, who are often trained via a White supremacist, anti-Black curriculum[8] may act on their own biases and forget that Black youth have strengths, show resilience, and have ample protective factors that support them through structural racism and racism-related stress. Researchers have highlighted various protective factors that influence the pathways from structural racism to racial health inequities, such as having Black collective spaces, digital activism, critical media literacy, strong racial identity, and social support.[8,15,16]

Assessing for and Documenting Historical Context and Protective Factors

Adolescent health providers are well positioned to not only assess for risk factors and the negative impact of anti-Black racism[17] but also to explore strengths, resilience, and protective factors that Black youth embody.[18] For example, Herbst and colleagues[19] offer a clinical framework for dismantling anti-Black racism by sensitizing providers to historical and contextual factors informing experiences with anti-Black racism and offering strategies to address anti-Black racism in clinical care. Providers can go a step further by using systems-centered language[20] to describe the role of anti-Black systemic racism on Black youth's health and health behaviors. Akin to person-first language (where the person is put before the disease), systems-centered language labels the intergenerational systems driving oppression and racism so that the humanity of those impacted by these anti-Black systems is upheld.[21] See **Box 2** for example. By contextualizing Black youth experiences within the clinical record, the harms of stereotyping and bias (ie, assuming a patient is non-adherent by

---

Box 2
Recommendations for systems-centered language in clinical context

Write:	Instead of:
"Patient X is a 15-year-old boy presenting with poor medication adherence due to exposure to financial barriers that drive his risk for type 2 diabetes."	*"Patient X is a 15-year-old Black boy presenting with poor medication adherence and at risk for type 2 diabetes"*

choice rather than considering the myriad structural barriers that prevent the youth from following the providers instructions) would be directly addressed. Pieterse and colleagues[22] also highlight other specific strategies that health service providers can apply to address racial trauma, such as cultural humility, empathic validation, empowerment strategies, and professional activism. Overall, the contextualization of risk with protective factors, structural competency,[23] and documenting the historical context for health behaviors are key strategies to ensure that anti-Black stereotypes and biases are addressed and eradicated within pediatric care settings.

Heteronormativity, Sexism, and Transphobia in Adolescent Health and Pediatric Care

Mirroring experiences of other historically oppressed populations, lesbian, gay, bisexual, transgender, non-binary, queer, questioning, asexual, or intersex (LGBTQ+) youth experience discrimination within medical and mental health settings.[24] One contributing factor to stigma in health care settings is the history of the diagnosis of homosexuality, which was removed from the Diagnostic and Statistical Manual of Mental Disorders-II in 1973 and from the International Classification of Diseases10 in 1992. Yet diagnoses concerning gender identity persist. Despite the prevailing stance against conversion therapy by every major pediatric and mental health professional association, many LGBTQ+ young people will experience pressure from a licensed health care professional to convert or change their sexual orientation and/or gender identity to meet heteronormativity and cisnormativity standards before they are 18 year old.[25,26] Acting on their own heterosexist and transphobic stigmatized views of LGBTQ+ people, which are further promulgated by major gaps in health professional curricula that fail to address these biases, health care professionals may pathologize LGBTQ+ people's sexual orientation and gender identity.[27–29] Thus, adolescent health providers must be equipped with knowledge and skills to promote trust among LGBTQ+ young people.[30,31] For example, providers must recognize that LGBTQ+ young people may have a history of discrimination when interacting with people they should be able to trust (eg, caregivers, health care providers).[25,32] Accordingly, providers should follow guidance from LGBTQ+ young people on how best to provide affirming care.[33,34]

LGBTQ+ young people present with elevated rates of mental and physical health problems, including higher rates of substance misuse and suicidal ideation and attempts.[35–37] These mental and physical health problems are linked with LGBTQ+ young people experiencing increased levels of heterosexism, transphobia, sexism, stigma, discrimination, and victimization.[37] Perhaps the most pernicious culprits of psychological harm to LGBTQ+ young people are sexual orientation[32,38] and gender identity[39,40] change efforts. These experiences reflect stigma, bias, and miseducation[41] which persist among health professionals, despite seminal research demonstrating that psychosocial functioning is improved for transgender and gender diverse youth who take gender-affirming hormones.[42]

INTERSECTIONALITY OF BLACK AND LESBIAN, GAY, BISEXUAL, TRANSGENDER, NON-BINARY, QUEER, QUESTIONING, ASEXUAL, OR INTERSEX YOUNG PEOPLE IN ADOLESCENT HEALTH

Increasing knowledge and practice of intersectionality within the field of adolescent health research and clinical practice is of utmost importance. By omitting conversations about intersectionality, the field of adolescent health—in research and practice—is missing half the story when it comes to critical examination of racism, heterosexism, and transphobia. Within an anti-racist praxis of meeting the mental health needs of young people presenting to pediatric care settings, other intersectional identities like gender identity, class, disability, and sexual orientation must be considered.[43] The intersectionality framework considers how multiple overlapping social identities contribute to social power and expression experienced by an individual or group.[43,44] Without consideration of multiple social identities, practitioners may overlook important influences on a patient's physical and mental health[45] such as the amplified role of mental health stigma from black communities and LGBTQ+ communities, preventing individuals from seeking care even when they desperately need it.[46] Such oversight could result in misdiagnosis and poorer treatment and health outcomes.[47] Professionals in the health care field need to recognize that intersectional identities translate to distinctly different experiences, which can further vary by context. For example, experiences in clinical care and mental health presentation may differ for a Latine heterosexual cisgender man versus a Black gay, nonbinary person. Intersectionality allows for the consideration of these nuanced experiences because it goes beyond checking category boxes to understanding how one's cultural identity as a racialized person enhances the marginalization or lack of community one experiences as a person of color with a sexual identity that is not accepted within their racialized community and how such rejection/acceptance might afford unique risks or protections over time.

ADOLESCENT HEALTH CARE PROMOTION IN THE POST-CORONAVIRUS DISEASE ERA

Following the peak of the COVID-19 pandemic, it became quite clear to health care providers that available approaches used to support adolescent health prior to the pandemic would not be sufficient. During the first 10 months of the COVID-19 pandemic, Black youth had a significant increase in suicide deaths.[48] A systematic review of the mental health impacts of COVID-19 on youth revealed an interconnection between caregiver and youth mental health, including increased levels of stress, anxiety, and depression among youth which varied by age, gender, race, ethnicity, socioeconomic status, and previous mental health or disability diagnosis.[49] A rapid review by Zolopa and colleagues[50] also revealed negative impacts of the pandemic on youth overall mental health.

Notably, youth appeared to gain important support services from schools prior to the pandemic. A study of acute mental health care utilization in United States children's hospitals before and after statewide COVID-19 school closure orders revealed that suicide or self-injury and depressive disorders drove increases in acute encounters in 44 United States children's hospitals after COVID-19–related school closures.[51] As we emerge into the post-COVID era, the urgent need for tailored and empowering multi-systemic resources for Black and LGBTQ + adolescents is fundamental.[52,53] Adolescent health care professionals are uniquely positioned to address anti-Black racism, heterosexism, and transphobia because they are frontline workers who may interact with youth when they are most vulnerable. In this post-COVID 19 era, where the systematic impact of health inequities have been made bare, it is imperative that adolescent health providers are guided by a health equity lens, and thus, engage in a process of detection, understanding, and reduction/elimination of health disparities.[54] Accordingly, the authors have adapted these elements into this health-equity adapted STYLE framework.

Framework for Addressing Anti-Black Racism, Heterosexism, and Transphobia

Amidst the various calls for action to address anti-Black racism,[55,56] the authors offer a framework for adolescent health providers to address issues of structural anti-Black

> **Box 3**
> **The self-examination, talk, yield time and space to learn from youth, learn about intersectionality and health inequity, evaluate policies and practices (STYLE) framework**
>
> Self-examination and critical reflection to improve awareness and understand personal experiences of oppression, privilege, biases, and reasons for inaction;
>
> Talk directly about anti-Black racism, heterosexism, and transphobia;
>
> Yield time and space to learn from Black LGBTQ+ youth about their health and wellbeing experiences;
>
> Learn about how intersectional racism, heterosexism, and transphobia drive health inequities;
>
> Evaluate policies and practice through an anti-Black racism, anti-heterosexism, and anti-transphobia lens.

racism, heterosexism, and transphobia using an equity lens. The authors adapted the STYLE framework[57,58] to consider health equity while addressing anti-Black racism, heterosexism, and transphobia praxis among adolescent health professionals in clinical care, academic, and advocacy settings. In brief, the health-equity adapted STYLE framework references 5 sets of practices that can be employed to promote health equity (**Box 3**).

Through the incorporation of the health-equity adapted STYLE framework (**Fig. 1**), adolescent health researchers and clinicians can address key intersectional identifiers in pediatric care settings. By adopting the health-equity adapted STYLE principles, adolescent health care researchers and practitioners can join the fight to dismantle systemic oppressive practices that negatively impact Black and LGBTQ+ adolescents.

As shown in **Table 1**, the authors adapted the STYLE framework[57,58] to promote the detection, understanding, and elimination/reduction of health disparities consistent with Kilbourne and colleague's model.[54] Specifically, Kilbourne and colleagues[54] developed a conceptual framework for understanding health disparities within a health care system. In this model, they describe 3 steps. The first step involves measuring disparities in poor health outcomes among populations made vulnerable by systemic racism/heterosexism/transphobia. The second step involves identification of determinants of health disparities at multiple levels of patient, provider, clinical encounter, and health care system. The third step is intervening to reduce/eliminate disparities and change policy around individual beliefs and preferences, effective patient-provider

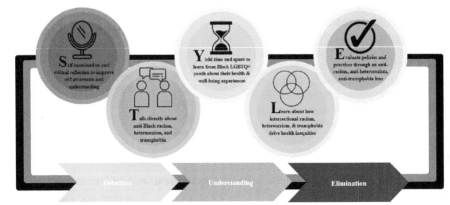

Fig. 1. The adapted STYLE health equity framework.

Table 1
Application of the adapted STYLE equity framework to address racism, heterosexism, and transphobia among Black and lesbian, gay, bisexual, transgender, non-binary, queer, questioning, asexual, or intersex adolescents

STYLE Framework	Detection	Understanding	Reduction/Elimination
Self-examination and critical reflection to improve awareness and understand personal experiences of oppression, privilege, biases, and reasons for inaction	Explore your knowledge and lived experiences and where gaps exist in working with Black and lesbian, gay, bisexual, transgender, non-binary, queer, questioning, asexual, or intersex (LGBTQ+) youth and families	Identify why the gaps exist in your knowledge and experiences and explore your reasons for inaction	Select 1–2 gaps to work on at a time and practice cultural humility[a] by committing to addressing the identified gaps over time
Talk directly about anti-Black racism, heterosexism, and transphobia	Examine areas in your current work to have discussions about anti-Black racism, heterosexism, and transphobia	Explore the barriers that get in the way of talking about these issues with colleagues, youth, and families	Find trusted colleagues and friends with whom you can have these conversations; as confidence builds, broach these topics with youth and families
Yield time and space to learn from Black LGBTQ+ youth about their health and wellbeing experiences	Identify opportunities to connect with, learn from, and support Black and LGBTQ+ youth	Examine barriers at patient, provider, clinical encounter, and health care system levels that get in the way of centering Black LGBTQ+ youth lived experiences	Build time into your clinical encounters, academic, recreational, and voluntary experiences to listen to the lived experience of Black LGBTQ+ youth
Learn about how intersectional racism, heterosexism, and transphobia drive health inequities	Expand your knowledge base about the specific race, gender, and sexual orientation disparities that occur for the health conditions you see in your clinics/hospital	Identify the systems level drivers of health disparities for those health conditions among Black and LGBTQ+ youth	Engage in didactic and experiential learning to increase awareness about how health disparities are sustained in Black and LGBTQ+ youth. Identify 1–2 ways you can contribute to dismantling these systemic inequities

(continued on next page)

Table 1
(continued)

STYLE Framework	Detection	Understanding	Reduction/Elimination
Evaluate policies and practices through an anti-Black racism, anti-heterosexism, and anti-transphobia lens	Identify divisional, departmental, and institutional policies and practices that uphold anti-Black racism, heterosexism, and transphobia	Understand why those policies exist by being curious and asking questions to administrators and leaders; identify allies who can help change those policies and practices	Advocate for policy and practice changes that will reduce anti-Black racism, heterosexism, and transphobia; promote the adoption of a health equity lens in decision-making by considering the needs of those most marginalized; support changes that are youth informed; seek out opportunities to change policies beyond your work setting, such as in local schools and communities

[a] Cultural humility involves the practice of: (i) lifelong learning and critical self-reflection, (ii) recognizing and challenging power imbalances via reflective listening and community-based research and advocacy, and (iii) institutional accountability.

communication, and organizational culture of the health care system. The authors adapted these elements into the STYLE framework (see **Table 1** for details). In the sections that follow, the authors situate the health-equity adapted STYLE framework within the context of clinical work via case studies.

Case Studies

In the following paragraphs are 3 case examples illustrating how the health-equity adapted STYLE framework can be used to promote an anti-racist, anti-heterosexist, and anti-transphobic clinical encounter.

Case 1 Title: Too feminine to be non-binary

Case Presentation: A biracial (Black/White) nonbinary adolescent was assigned female at birth but began to question their identity in middle school. Within a short timeframe, they realized their nonbinary identity and disclosed it to their parents which also coincided with starting at an all-female private school. The school and staff accommodated the adolescent's non-legal name and pronouns in emails and class rosters. However, they did not make accommodations for the traditionally female presenting uniform. This resulted in some incongruence with the adolescent's identity and led to some mental health challenges. Similarly, the adolescent's parents wanted to be accepting but their father was more passive in his acceptance and deferred to his wife. Their Black mother was not convinced that her child was nonbinary. In particular, the mother felt this way because her adolescent had always presented as "too feminine" to be nonbinary. Thus, the mother struggled to support her child's gender identity expression, especially the use of a binder.

Case Study 1: Clinical Questions

1. What role can adolescent health clinicians and researchers play in increasing knowledge about nonbinary gender identity for families, as these individuals may not be seen in gender clinics?

2. How might the adolescent's biracial identity contribute to the dynamic of their parent's understanding and acceptance of their child as nonbinary? What role can adolescent health care providers play in helping families understand, accept, and support youth in this situation?

3. How can adolescent health clinicians and researchers promote changing and adopting school policies and practices that support gender diverse students, namely single gender schools and schools with uniforms

---

Case Study 1: Discussion using STYLE framework within clinical context

Self-examination: Clinicians would be better informed about the intersectional stigma this patient is experiencing if they have reflected on their own gender and race intersectional privileges, and if through that reflection they have become aware of their knowledge gaps and stereotypes about biracial identity and gender nonconformity.

Talk: Clinicians would engage in a discussion with caregivers about the co-occurring stigmas of anti-Black racism and transphobia with an emphasis on nonbinary identity. Clinicians would emphasize to caregivers the necessity of validating their child's intersecting identities in order to protect and support their mental and physical health.

Yield time and space to learn from youth: Clinicians would intentionally create space during their provider-patient interaction to ask questions and listen to the lived experience of this biracial nonbinary youth to better understand their needs and inform their care.

Learn about intersectionality and health inequity: Clinicians would read articles, listen to talks, and attend community events to gain a deeper understanding of how anti-Black racism and transphobia (specific to nonbinary gender identity) can uniquely interact to impact bias, stigma, and discrimination. Clinicians would situate their learnings about intersectional stigma into the context of differential health outcomes for these youth.

Evaluate policies and practices: Clinicians would evaluate the direct and indirect impact of policies that force nonbinary biracial youth to conform (ie, identify a certain way, dress a certain way) on academic performance, mental health, and physical health. Clinicians would also evaluate how school policies can be informed by adolescent health research to better serve youth with multiple marginalized intersectional identities.

Case 2 Title: Parental gatekeeping and provider bias.

Case Presentation: In order to start hormone therapy, a Black transgender adolescent girl was required by her mother to disclose her gender identity (ie, "come out") to her father. The client's parents were not living together and had no communication with each other. The adolescent was worried that her father—who held some custodial rights—would deny her the ability to start hormonal therapy. The adolescent's worries were driven by her father's occupation as a rapper whose musical lyrics included misogynistic, homophobic, and transphobic language. Months of preparation via role-playing in therapy culminated in a session with the adolescent and her father. When she came out during the session, her father accepted her gender identity. The client was elated at the ability to start hormones. The scheduled gender clinic appointment was canceled by the adolescent's mother and the mother pulled the adolescent from therapy. Perhaps the mother did not expect the adolescent to disclose her identity or expected the father to be unsupportive of his child's gender identity and transition, including her desire for hormonal therapy. Ultimately, the client's mother engaged in medical gatekeeping.

Case Study 2: Clinical Questions

1. How did bias over the father's public persona complicate the clinical picture for the clinician and within the family?

2. Should the clinician have discussed the possibility with the mother and client that the client's parents first communicate amongst themselves?

3. What are ways to assess for caregiver medical gatekeeping especially when it comes to gender health?

Case Study 2: Discussion using STYLE framework within clinical context

Self-examination: Clinicians should engage in critical self-reflection to examine their own biases. For example, there was an assumption or bias by the clinician that the mother was more open and honest given her job as a school administrator rather than the father who performs songs with misogynistic, heterosexist, and transphobic lyrics. Instead, the clinician can use self-examination to consider that a public persona may not be a full representation of a caregiver's behavior. Clinicians should examine their barriers to working effectively with people who hold different value systems through an anti-Black racist, anti-heterosexist, and anti-transphobic lens.

Talk: Proactively engage with all caregivers (ensuring the adolescent is also involved in such conversations) about how they can best support their child; define and discuss medical gatekeeping and associated mental and physical health consequences.

Yield time and space to learn from youth: Clinicians should create space to hear about the lived experiences of Black transgender youth and how layers of their identities are and are not accepted within their communities.

Learn about intersectionality and health inequity: Clinicians should intentionally engage in learning experiences that deepen their knowledge of how intersectional racism and transphobia affect adolescents' health outcomes, engagement with health care providers, and reception of support from family and community members.

Evaluate policies and practices: Clinicians should explore how medical gatekeeping policies and practices directly and indirectly influence adolescent health. Clinicians should understand the short-term and long-term implications of delayed hormone therapy initiation on Black transgender youth and advocate for youth to reduce negative health outcomes.

Case 3 Title: Racism versus heterosexism; intersectionality means both

Case Presentation: A Black cisgender transracial adopted adolescent girl identifying as omnisexual (ie, attracted to more than 1 gender) was referred for therapy by her 2 White mothers for anxiety, depression, suicidal thoughts, and peer teasing. She was a highly capable student whose grades did not always reflect her abilities. She was enrolled in a prestigious language immersion private school where she was the only Black student. Upon further inquiry, the adolescent disclosed that the teasing she experienced was often race-based and caused racial trauma. At the time, the adolescent was not well informed on her biological historical heritage. She also had not been open with her parents about the extent of the racially motivated victimization as she did not realize that what she was experiencing was racial trauma. When she complained about other kids being mean to her, her mothers told her to "just ignore it."

Case Study 3: Clinical Questions

1. How might the mothers' White lesbian identities obscure the provider's understanding of the adolescent's ethnoracial and gender identity stages?

2. What are the factors to consider for a White clinician educating a Black adolescent on racial identity and racial trauma?

3. What kinds of responsibility are needed for transracial adoptive parents to teach their children about their biological heritage?

Case Study 3: Discussion using STYLE framework within clinical context

Self-examination: Clinicians critically examine their own biases and gaps in awareness about transracial adoptions of Black children by White LGBTQ+ parents (eg, assumptions that members of one minoritized group [lesbian women] will be equipped to discuss experiences of another minoritized group [Black adolescents]).

Talk: Clinicians engage in conversations with the family about the protective effects of ethnic identity and how empowering understanding one's historical heritage can be for transracial adoptees. Clinicians talk to families about the toll of racial trauma and heterosexism on academic performance, mental health, and physical health.

Yield time and space to learn from youth: Clinicians protect time during the clinical encounter to learn from adolescents about the nuances of their experiences with peer victimization. Reflective listening can help label experiences for young people who may not be aware of the layers of racial trauma.

Learn about intersectionality and health inequity: By engaging in didactics and independent learning, clinicians can build their knowledge of the complexities of transracial adoption, racial trauma, and heterosexism; advance their understanding of how factors associated with these intersectional identities drive health inequities; and engage in evidence-based strategies to reduce negative impacts on adolescents and families.

Evaluate policies and practices: Clinicians should advocate and partner with caregivers and youth to ensure that schools have policies that promote belonging and equity, address peer victimization (including racialized bullying) when it occurs, and intentionally create an environment where racial bigotry and heterosexism is not tolerated.

CLINICS CARE POINTS: EVIDENCE-BASED PEARLS

- Culturally Humble Care: Embrace humble curiosity and ongoing commitment[59] to learning about the lived experience of Black LGBTQ+ youth and understanding how their experiences impact health and well-being, recognizing that the experiences of youth from marginalized racial, sexual, and gender identity groups vary significantly.[8] Implement strategies to identify and address bias among adolescent health care providers.

- Education and Awareness: Implement educational programs and awareness campaigns that address racism, heterosexism, and transphobia within clinics, schools, and institutions.[3,9] Have readily available resources for adolescents and families to help them recognize and combat the various forms of discrimination.

- Safe Spaces: Create safe and inclusive health care environments where adolescents feel seen and heard and are comfortable discussing their lived experiences with racism, heterosexism, and transphobia.[31]

- Intersectionality: Recognize and address the intersection of multiple identities, such as race, gender, and sexual orientation, to better understand the unique challenges faced by adolescents at these intersections.[45,46]

- Community Engagement: Collaborate with community organizations and activist groups to promote anti-racist, LGBTQ+ affirming, and inclusive practices that extend beyond research and clinical settings.

CLINICS CARE POINTS: EVIDENCE-BASED PITFALLS

- Assuming Homogeneity: Avoid assuming that all adolescents from a particular racial, sexual, or gender identity group have the same experiences or needs.[60] Recognize the diversity within the communities of adolescents with these identities.

- Failure to Update Practices: Be aware of changing terminology and evolving best practices in detecting, understanding, and addressing racism, heterosexism, and transphobia. Failing to update clinical and research practices can result in use of outdated and ineffective interventions and research methods.[24]

- Tokenism: Avoid tokenistic efforts, such as featuring a single representative from a marginalized group in promotional materials. Such practices can be seen as insincere and insufficient in addressing health inequities.[61]

- Neglecting Mental Health: Be mindful of the mental health consequences of racism, heterosexism, and transphobia on adolescents and their families.[45] Ensure that support for mental health is an integral part of any adolescent health promotion strategy.
- Ignoring Feedback: Listen to the lived experiences of adolescents, their families, and communities regarding the effectiveness and impact of anti-racist, LGBTQ+ affirming, and inclusive effort.[62] Failure to heed their input can lead to missed opportunities for improvement or worse yet implementation of strategies that unintentionally cause harm and increase health inequities.

DISCLOSURE

The authors have nothing to disclose.

REFERENCES

1. Williams DR, Lawrence JA, Davis BA. Racism and health: evidence and needed research. Annu Rev Publ Health 2019;40:105–25.
2. Alegría M, NeMoyer A, Falgàs Bagué I, et al. Social determinants of mental health: Where we are and where we need to go. Curr Psychiatr Rep 2018;20:1–13.
3. Thurston IB, Alegría M, Hood KB, et al. How psychologists can help achieve equity in health care—advancing innovative partnerships and models of care delivery: Introduction to the special issue. Am Psychol 2023;78(2):73–81.
4. Smedley BD. The lived experience of race and its health consequences. Am J Publ Health 2012;102(5):933–5.
5. Salami B, Idi Y, Anyieth Y, et al. Factors that contribute to the mental health of Black youth. Can Med Assoc J 2022;194(41):E1404–10.
6. Bonilla-Silva E. Rethinking racism: toward a structural interpretation. Am Socio Rev 1997;62(3):465–80.
7. Braun L. Theorizing race and racism: preliminary reflections on the medical curriculum. J Law Med 2017;43(2–3):239–56.
8. Volpe VV, Hoggard LS, Willis HA, et al. Anti-Black structural racism goes online: a conceptual model for racial health disparities research. Ethn Dis 2021;31(Suppl 1):311–8.
9. Woods-Jaeger B, Gaylord-Harden N, Dinizulu SM, et al. Developing practices for hospital-based violence intervention programs to address anti-Black racism and historical trauma. Am Psychol 2023;78(2):199–210.
10. Yusuf HE, Copeland-Linder N, Young AS, et al. The impact of racism on the health and wellbeing of black indigenous and other youth of color (BIPOC youth). Child and Adolescent Psychiatric Clinics of North America 2022;31(2):261–75.
11. Dumornay NM, Lebois LA, Ressler KJ, et al. Racial disparities in adversity during childhood and the false appearance of race-related differences in brain structure. Am J Psychiatr 2023;180(2):127–38.
12. Price MA, Weisz JR, McKetta S, et al. Are psychotherapies less effective for Black youth in communities with higher levels of anti-Black racism? J Am Acad Child Adolesc Psychiatr 2022;61(6):754–63.
13. Roulston C, McKetta S, Price M, et al. Structural correlates of mental health support access among sexual minority youth of color during COVID-19. J Clin Child Adolesc Psychol 2022;52(5):649–58.
14. Adichie CN. The danger of a single story. Video. TEDGlobal, Available at: https://www.ted.com/talks/chimamanda_ngozi_adichie_the_danger_of_a_single_story, 2009. Accessed February 26, 2024.

15. King L. The media and Black masculinity: Looking at the media through race[d] lenses. Crit Educ 2017;8(2):31–40.
16. Attachment perspectives on race, prejudice, and anti-racism: Introduction to the Special Issue. In: Stern JA, Barbarin O, Cassidy J, editors. Am J Bioeth 2022; 24(3):253–9.
17. Chung EK, Siegel BS, Garg A, et al. Screening for social determinants of health among children and families living in poverty: A guide for clinicians. Curr Probl Pediatr Adolesc Health Care 2016;46(5):135–53.
18. Murry VM, Butler-Barnes ST, Mayo-Gamble TL, et al. Excavating new constructs for family stress theories in the context of everyday life experiences of Black American families. Journal of Family Theory & Review 2018;10(2):384–405.
19. Herbst R, Corley AM, McTate E. Clinical Framework for dismantling Antiblack racism in the clinic room. Clin Pediatr 2023;62(10):1129–36.
20. O'Reilly M. Systems centered language: Speaking truth to power during COVID-19 while confronting racism, Available at: https://meagoreillyphd.medium.com/systems-centered-language-a3dc7951570e. Accessed February 26, 2024.
21. Buchanan NT, Perez M, Prinstein MJ, et al. Upending racism in psychological science: Strategies to change how science is conducted, reported, reviewed, and disseminated. Am Psychol 2021;76(7):1097–112.
22. Pieterse AL, Austin CL, Nicolas AI, et al. Essential elements for working with racial trauma: A guide for health service psychologists. Prof Psychol Res Pract 2023; 54(3):213–20.
23. Wang EE. Structural competency: What Is It, why do we need it, and what does the structurally competent emergency physician look like? AEM education and training 2019;4(1):S140–2.
24. Ker A, Gardiner T, Carroll R, et al. "We just want to be treated normally and to have that healthcare that comes along with it": Rainbow young people's experiences of primary care in Aotearoa New Zealand. Youth 2022;2(4):691–704.
25. Mallory C, Brown TNT, Conron KJ. Conversion therapy and LGBT youth. Los Angeles, CA: UCLA School of Law Williams Institute; 2019.
26. SAMHSA, Moving beyond change efforts: Evidence and action to support and affirm LGBTQI+ Youth, Available at: https://store.samhsa.gov/sites/default/files/pep22-03-12-001.pdf, 2023. Accessed February 26, 2024.
27. Lothwell LE, Libby N, Adelson SL. Mental health care for LGBT youths. Focus 2020;18(3):268–76.
28. Riggs DW, Ansara YG, Treharne GJ. An evidence-based model for understanding the mental health experiences of transgender Australians. Aust Psychol 2015; 50(1):32–9.
29. Tan KK, Schmidt JM, Ellis SJ, et al. 'It's how the world around you treats you for being trans': mental health and wellbeing of transgender people in Aotearoa New Zealand. Psychology & Sexuality 2022;13(5):1109–21.
30. Adelson SL. of Child TAA. Practice parameter on gay, lesbian, or bisexual sexual orientation, gender nonconformity, and gender discordance in children and adolescents. J Am Acad Child Adolesc Psychiatr 2012;51(9):957–74.
31. Fields EL. Achieving health equity for sexual and gender-diverse youth. Pediatric Clinics 2023;70(4):813–35.
32. Ryan C, Toomey RB, Diaz RM, et al. Parent-initiated sexual orientation change efforts with LGBT adolescents: Implications for young adult mental health and adjustment. J Homosex 2020;67(2):159–73.

33. Fraser G, Brady A, Wilson MS. Mental health support experiences of rainbow rangatahi youth in Aotearoa New Zealand: results from a co-designed online survey. J Roy Soc N Z 2022;52(4):472–89.
34. Bowen S, Ker A, McLeod KE, et al. Messages from rainbow rangatahi to mental health professionals in training. Kotuitui: New Zealand Journal of Social Sciences 2023;1–21.
35. De Lange J, Baams L, Van Bergen DD, et al. Minority stress and suicidal ideation and suicide attempts among LGBT adolescents and young adults: A meta-analysis. LGBT Health 2022;9(4):222–37.
36. Plöderl M, Tremblay P. Mental health of sexual minorities. A systematic review. Int Rev Psychiatr 2015;27(5):367–85.
37. Wilson C, Cariola LA. LGBTQI+ youth and mental health: A systematic review of qualitative research. Adolescent Research Review. 2020;5:187–211.
38. Chan RC, Leung JSY, Wong DCK. Experiences, motivations, and impacts of sexual orientation change efforts: Effects on sexual identity distress and mental health among sexual minorities. Sex Res Soc Pol 2022;1–15.
39. Fenaughty J, Tan K, Ker A, et al. Sexual orientation and gender identity change efforts for young people in New Zealand: Demographics, types of suggesters, and associations with mental health. J Youth Adolesc 2023;52(1):149–64.
40. Turban JL, King D, Reisner SL, et al. Psychological attempts to change a person's gender identity from transgender to cisgender: Estimated prevalence across US States, 2015. Am J Publ Health 2019;109(10):1452–4.
41. Green AE, Price-Feeney M, Dorison SH, et al. Self-reported conversion efforts and suicidality among US LGBTQ youths and young adults, 2018. Am J Publ Health 2020;110(8):1221–7.
42. Chen D, Berona J, Chan YM, et al. Psychosocial functioning in transgender youth after 2 years of hormones. N Engl J Med 2023;388(3).
43. Crenshaw KW. Demarginalizing the intersection of race and sex: A Black feminist critique of antidiscrimination doctrine, feminist theory and antiracist politics, *Univ Chicago Leg Forum*, 139 (1), 1989, Article 8. Available at: https://chicagounbound. uchicago.edu/uclf/vol1989/iss1/8. Accessed February 26, 2024.
44. Bowleg L. The problem with the phrase women and minorities: Intersectionality—an important theoretical framework for public health. Am J Publ Health 2012;102(7): 1267–73.
45. Fagrell Trygg N, Gustafsson PE, Månsdotter A. Languishing in the crossroad? A scoping review of intersectional inequalities in mental health. Int J Equity Health 2019;18(1):1–13.
46. DuPont-Reyes MJ, Villatoro AP, Phelan JC, et al. Adolescent views of mental illness stigma: An intersectional lens. Am J Orthopsychiatry 2020;90(2):201–11.
47. Miller HL, Thomi M, Patterson RM, et al. Effects of intersectionality along the pathway to diagnosis for autistic children with and without co-occurring attention deficit hyperactivity disorder in a nationally-representative sample. J Autism Dev Disord 2022;53(9):3542–57.
48. Bridge JA, Ruch DA, Sheftall AH, et al. Youth suicide during the first year of the COVID-19 pandemic. Pediatrics 2023;151(3). e2022058375.
49. Naff D, Williams S, Furman-Darby J, et al. The mental health impacts of COVID-19 on PK–12 students: A systematic review of emerging literature. AERA Open 2022. https://doi.org/10.1177/23328584221084722.
50. Zolopa C, Burack JA, O'Connor RM, et al. Changes in youth mental health, psychological wellbeing, and substance use during the COVID-19 pandemic: A rapid review. Adolescent Research Review 2022;7(2):161–77.

51. Zima BT, Edgcomb JB, Rodean J, et al. Use of acute mental health care in US children's hospitals before and after statewide COVID-19 school closure orders. Psychiatr Serv 2022;73(11):1202–9.
52. Bogan E, Adams-Bass VN, Francis LA, et al. "Wearing a mask won't protect us from our history": The impact of COVID-19 on Black children and families. Soc Pol Rep 2022;35(2):1–33.
53. Fish JN, McInroy LB, Paceley MS, et al. "I'm kinda stuck at home with unsupportive parents right now": LGBTQ youths' experiences with COVID-19 and the importance of online support. J Adolesc Health 2020;67(3):450–2.
54. Kilbourne AM, Switzer G, Hyman K, et al. Advancing health disparities research within the health care system: A conceptual framework. Am J Publ Health 2006; 96(12):2113–21.
55. Cheung CK, Tucker-Seeley R, Davies S, et al. A call to action: Antiracist patient engagement in adolescent and young adult oncology research and advocacy. Future Oncol 2021;17(28):3743–56.
56. Jindal M, Heard-Garris N, Empey A, et al. Getting "our house" in order: Re-building academic pediatrics by dismantling the Anti-Black Racist Foundation. Academic Pediatrics 2020;20(8):1044–50.
57. Fix RL, Testa EG, Thurston IB, et al. Anti-racism strategies in pediatric psychology: Using STYLE can help children overcome adverse experiences with police. J Clin Psychol Med Settings 2022;29(2):262–73.
58. Fix RL, Thurston IB, Johnson RM, et al. Promoting anti-racism in the legal system: An application of the STYLE framework. Front Psychol 2023;14:1061637.
59. Tervalon M, Murray-Garcia J. Cultural humility versus cultural competence: A critical distinction in defining physician training outcomes in multicultural education. J Health Care Poor Underserved 1998;9(2):117–25.
60. Eberhardt JL. Biased: Uncovering the hidden prejudice that shapes what we see, think, and do. Penguin. 2020. Available at: https://www.penguinrandomhouse.com/books/557462/biased-by-jennifer-l-eberhardt-phd/. [Accessed 22 February 2024].
61. Arunkumar K, Bowman DD, Coen SE, et al. Conceptualizing youth participation in children's health research: Insights from a youth-driven process for developing a youth advisory council. Children 2018;6(1):3.
62. Jadwin-Cakmak L, Bauermeister JA, Cutler JM, et al. The Health Access Initiative: A training and technical assistance program to improve health care for sexual and gender minority youth. J Adolesc Health 2020;67(1):115–22.

Moving?

Make sure your subscription moves with you!

To notify us of your new address, find your **Clinics Account Number** (located on your mailing label above your name), and contact customer service at:

Email: journalscustomerservice-usa@elsevier.com

800-654-2452 (subscribers in the U.S. & Canada)
314-447-8871 (subscribers outside of the U.S. & Canada)

Fax number: 314-447-8029

Elsevier Health Sciences Division
Subscription Customer Service
3251 Riverport Lane
Maryland Heights, MO 63043

*To ensure uninterrupted delivery of your subscription, please notify us at least 4 weeks in advance of move.

Printed and bound by CPI Group (UK) Ltd, Croydon, CR0 4YY

08/05/2025

01864724-0001